KETO DIET COOKBOOK AFTER 50:

Eat the Food You Love and Stay Healthy.
A Complete Guide with Over 250 Simple Recipes to
Balance Hormones, Lose Weight, and Regain Your
Metabolism. For Women and Men.

AMY CONTESSA

TABLE OF CONTENTS

Introduction

Keto diet is essentially a high-fat, exceptionally low-carb diet. It was first introduced in the 1920s as a way for people to lose weight. The Ketogenic diet has also been dubbed as 'Atkins on steroids'. Ketogenic diet involves eating 5-10% of calories from carbohydrates, 20-30% protein, and 65-75% fat, and then cutting all carbohydrate-containing foods. A keto dieter's body then goes into a metabolic state known as ketosis, which helps in burning fat.

One can start this diet only after consulting a certified doctor initially. He would then plan out a keto diet.

The high-fat keto diet promotes an increase in ketone production, as the body finds the ketones to be a more efficient energy source. During ketosis, one's body switches from burning carbohydrates to burning fats. The body starts burning the fat which is stored in the body. So, it is a diet for weight loss.

The Ketogenic diet contains a lot of foods, which help the body reduce its cholesterol levels and control blood sugar levels. The diet also focuses on electrolyte ratio and increases the intake of fiber. The keto diet cuts down on carbs, as they take longer to digest. This diet also helps one to lose excess water weight. It results in rapid fat loss.

Since the diet focuses on increasing the intake of fats and proteins, there is little chance for food being converted into sugar. The lack of carbs in the diet can lead to mood swings and dizziness at first. If one begins eating less carbs, their brain gets less carbs which can lead to them feeling less happy.

The keto diet has many benefits to the body, it is linked to lower cholesterol and blood pressure and also lowers triglycerides. It also controls blood sugar and reduces the risk of many cancers. It also helps the body to release fatty acids from the adipose tissues. This helps in preventing inflammation, stabilizing blood sugar levels, improving heart health and lowering the risk of diabetes.

It also has the ability to regenerate brain cells.. The keto diet helps in maintaining lean muscle mass. It also promotes a hormonal stabilization, as well as strength and stamina. However, it is also said that a long term keto diet can cause kidney damage. It can also cause gallstones development. Too much saturated fats can also cause high cholesterol levels.

The keto diet is an excellent diet which helps the body to shed weight much faster when compared to the Atkins diet. The only concern for this diet is that it is difficult for the brain to get used to long term carbohydrates starvation. Most of the dieticians recommend a keto diet to be followed for only short periods of time. Not only does this diet help in weight loss, but also enhances the athletic performance, helps in increased energy levels and also improves brain health.

The ketogenic diet is an excellent diet which can help in weight loss. It is also a good option for people who have diabetes. It is a diet which has been used for over a century. However, it has been disregarded for decades, and now it is slowly gaining popularity. People have been looking for a diet which promises high quality food and help them lose weight. The keto diet is the best option for such people . The diet does promise to help people lose weight and also build muscles. However, it is often detested because of its side effects. People do not want their physical appearance to change. However, good diets contain proteins and fats. The side effects of this diet are also unknown. Unlike other diets, after the initial stages of the diet, it is not necessary to take any medicines.

The ketogenic diet has a very low quantity of carbs in it. Therefore, the brain feels much less fatigue. Since the diet is high in fat, after the initial stages, the brain gets used to burning fats instead of carbs.

READ ON to find out more on keto diet and to learn new keto diet recipe that will help you live a healthy, slim and happy life.

CHAPTER 1:

The Keto Diet

Why Is It Important to Stick To The Ketogenic Meal Plan?

We have tackled this topic several times in this guidebook already. However, the question 'why is it important to stick to the Ketogenic diet' keeps coming up all the time. As we stated earlier, the Ketogenic diet has numerous benefits to you once you have decided to start on it. Let us find an answer to this recurring question.

The Ketogenic diet is important because:

It reduces your blood's insulin and sugar levels

if you have diabetes, the Ketogenic diet is very helpful. Doing away with carbohydrates is proven to reduce your blood sugar levels drastically. This also reduces your insulin levels in the blood. This is, however, efficient if you have visited and consulted with your doctor, and they have suggested the Ketogenic meal plan for you. This diet could even remedy type 2 diabetes.

It lowers your body's blood pressure: Hypertension is a great risk factor to you because you could contact other diseases such as stroke, kidney failure, or even heart-related diseases. However, sticking to the Ketogenic diet could prove itself beneficial because doing away with carbohydrates lowers your blood pressure and thus reduces your chances of contracting the diseases mentioned above and could assist you in living longer.

It improves your LDL Cholesterol levels: If you have high LDL cholesterol levels, you stand a great risk of contracting heart-related diseases, including possible heart attacks. This depends on the particle size of the LD. If you have large particles, then your chances of suffering from a heart attack are low, while having small particles increases your risk of suffering from a possible heart attack. The Ketogenic diet increases the LDL particles in size in your blood. Thus, if you opt to lower your consumption of carbohydrates, you are improving your chances of avoiding a possible heart attack.

It is a therapy for brain disorders: Glucose is very important for your brain in its day to day functioning. Your brain burns glucose to provide energy for it to function normally. Once you adopt the Ketogenic diet, your body's liver is forced to produce glucose from the protein you ingest. However, your brain can also burn ketones, which are a result of the Ketogenic diet. This way, the diet remedies epilepsy in children who are unresponsive to the drugs related to epilepsy. The diet could be a possible cure for epilepsy. The diet is also known for its ability to remedy Alzheimer's disease as well as Parkinson's disease.

It lowers your body's triglycerides: If you are wondering what triglycerides are, they are fat molecules that move in your blood. It has been proven that high levels of triglycerides could lead to heart-related diseases. These levels are elevated in your body if you consume high amounts of carbohydrates, and thus, the diet comes in handy and assists you to cut on your carbs consumption. Additionally, consuming low fats could also raise the levels of triglycerides in your blood, which makes the Ketogenic diet appropriate to stick to.

This diet is an effective agent in your attempts to lose weight. You are cutting carbohydrates in your diet in the most effective way for you to lose weight. Low carb diets are very effective in weight loss because of their ability to get rid of excess water in your body in the process lowering your body's insulin levels, which in turn speeds up your weight loss. This is, however, effective in short-term weight loss and not so effective for the long-term plan. This is why it is important to seek your physician's opinion before embarking on the diet.

It reduces your appetite: The Ketogenic diet is important in reducing your appetite if you are trying to fight obesity. Hunger is what leads to overeating and becoming obese in the end. Cutting carbohydrates in your meal and ingesting more fats and proteins leads to consuming fewer calories. Doing away with carbohydrates is one way to minimize your appetite as well as your intake of calories.

If you are looking to boost your blood's sugar and insulin levels or if you are looking to lose appetite, lose weight, lower your triglycerides, remedying brain disorders, lowering your blood pressure or becoming healthier in general, you have all the reasons to stick to the diet.

How Long Would It Take for The Ketogenic Diet To Be Effective?

By now, you already know that the Ketogenic diet is among the world's famous low carbohydrates diet. The diet is responsible for the reason why your body no longer burns carbohydrates

instead, it burns fats to produce ketones that are responsible for the day to day functioning of your body. After adopting the diet, the question 'how long until you enter ketosis' begs for attention. Most people get worried that they might not enter ketosis in time, and thus, they tend to give up on a diet as a result.

The fact is that the amount of time it would take you to enter ketosis is not the same amount of time someone else could need to get into ketosis. Additionally, many people find it hard for their bodies to enter ketosis. Let us take a look at how long it could take you to enter ketosis.

For you to benefit from the diet, your body needs to get into ketosis first. Ketosis, as we defined it earlier, is a state that your body adapts to when it starts burning fats into molecules, which we referred to as ketones. Ketones are your body's main source of energy once your body stops burning carbohydrates to produce glucose, usually the main source of energy on the normal diet.

The first step that you would take as a way of reaching ketosis is doing away with carbohydrates. It is important to note that your body stores excess glucose in your liver or your muscles. The glucose is stored in its storage form, glycogen. Switching to burning fats by your body could take time because your body would be required to burn all the glucose in your body before opting to burn fats for energy. The time required for your body to successfully make this change is different from everyone else. This could be because of varying carbohydrates intake in your daily meals as well as varying consumptions of proteins, fats, or how regularly you exercise your body, your age, or even your body's metabolism rates.

For instance, if you consume carbohydrates at high or elevated levels, once you have started on the Ketogenic diet, your body could take longer before it gets into ketosis. This is contrary to your consumption of carbohydrates as an average or lower consumer. It would take you a shorter time compared to the high levels of carbohydrates consumers to get into ketosis. This is because your body would be required to finish all its glucose in the body, including the stored glycogen. The more carbohydrates you consume, the more the stored glycogen and the more the amount of time required to burn it in your body completely.

It would require you between 2 to 5 days, if you are an average consumer of carbohydrates, to get into ketosis. This is approximate if you consume 50 to 60 grams of carbohydrates in a day. The duration of time could be altered depending on several factors, including

the body's metabolism, your age, your level of physical activity as well as your protein, carbohydrates, and fat intake.

You would be able to tell if you are on ketosis if you experienced a number of symptoms, including the Ketogenic flu. You could experience nausea, bad breath, elevated thirst, or fatigue. These are possible ways to tell if you are already on ketosis. However, the most accurate and reliable source of knowledge on your ketosis level is if you test your body of the ketone levels. You could opt to visit your doctor or physician, and they would run a few tests on you to determine the ketone levels in your body. Or you could measure the Beta-hydroxybutyrate levels using the ketone meter at the comfort of your house.

Some people take longer to get into ketosis because they most probably ingest carbohydrates without knowing. Consuming carbohydrates could hinder the rate at which it would require your body to get into ketosis. It could as well get your body out of ketosis in the process. There is no standard limit to limit your consumption of carbohydrates to ensure that your body gets into ketosis. Different people could get into ketosis by eating different levels of carbohydrates you included. This is why it is important to consult with your doctor. Another possible reason could be that you are not ingesting the required levels of fats in your diet. The Ketogenic advocates for up to 70% of fats to be consumed as well as 20% of protein and possibly 5% or 10% of carbohydrates. Changing or altering this ratio could mean you will take longer to get into ketosis. Other reasons could be your age, physical exercise levels, personal stress, or even lack of adequate sleep. These could affect the rate at which your body could get into ketosis.

You could improve your chance of getting into ketosis if you exercise regularly, minimize your carbohydrates consumption, increase your fat consumption, or even by testing your ketone levels regularly.

CHAPTER 2:

Benefits Of Keto Diet After 50

There are a lot of benefits in starting a ketogenic diet, be it in terms of weight, experience or to improve your health!

Effective in fighting Epilepsy

The primary goal of this diet, introduced in Antiquity, was to fight against epilepsy. The ketones may affect anti-convulsion, but to date it is not possible to say why they have this effect on the body.

Without going too far into the scientific part, ketone bodies would have an impact on the concentrations of glutamate and GABA (Gamma-Amino Butyric Acid). Glutamate is the main excitatory neuromediator of the central nervous system and GABA the main inhibitory neuromediator. This would explain why the ketogenic diet has such important effects on people with epilepsy. But I don't want to lose you with my scientific explanations, you can do your own research if the subject interests you.

Effective in Weight Loss

Your body's source of energy in the ketogenic diet is fat, either from food or stored by your body. This therefore has advantages: the level of insulin, a hormone that stores fat, drops very significantly, this means that your body will become more efficient at burning fat.

Effective in Type I or Type II Diabetes

The diabetes results in a problem in the metabolism of carbohydrates, the diet is therefore naturally a place to relieve the signs and symptoms in a person with diabetes, whether for a type I or type II diabetes. In fact, whether the problem is a defect in insulin production or insulin resistance, the ketogenic diet will make it possible to get around the problem.When you are keto-adapted, your blood sugar drops sharply because you only eat foods low in carbohydrates. The ketogenic diet can therefore allow you to control your blood sugar, which can be very effective in managing your diabetes. The ketogenic diet will allow you to reduce your insulin levels to healthy and stable values.

Effective in People with Alzheimer's

Excuse me in advance, but in this part, we will tackle a scientific "hair" side to explain the benefits of the ketogenic diet in the treatment of Alzheimer's disease. The ketogenic diet is effective in the treatment of neurodegenerative diseases like Alzheimer because it aims to increase the enzymes of the mitochondrial metabolism. Clearly, this would develop more energy in the brain, and therefore improve cognitive efficiency. In addition to all this, the ketogenic diet would have a role in protecting against oxidative stress, and therefore would be preventive and effective against cell death. This would therefore limit brain degeneration.

Improves Concentration

The ketones are a very good source of fuel for the brain. As you decrease your carbohydrate intake, you avoid blood sugar spikes, which often appear after meals. This allows your body to avoid focusing on eliminating carbohydrates and to focus on the activity you are doing.

Good for Cholesterol

As said above, if you pay attention to the quality of the fats you consume, you will see an improvement in cholesterol: you will see your good cholesterol (HDL: High Density Lipoprotein) increase, while your bad cholesterol (LDL: Low Density Lipoprotein) will decrease.

You will also notice an improvement in triglyceride levels, as well as an improvement in blood pressure. Blood pressure problems are usually caused by being overweight, and the ketogenic diet is intended to cause weight loss and therefore reduce blood pressure problems.

Foods Allowed in Keto Diet

To make the most of your diet, there are prohibited foods, and others that are allowed, but in limited quantities. Here are the foods allowed in the ketogenic diet:

Food allowed in unlimited quantities

Lean or fatty meats

No matter which meat you choose, it contains no carbohydrates so thatthat you can have fun! Pay attention to the quality of your meat, and the amount of fat. Alternate between fatty meats and lean meats!

Here are some examples of lean meats:

Beef: sirloin steak, roast beef, 5% minced steak, roast, flank steak, tenderloin, grisons meat, tripe, kidneys

Horse: roti, steak

Pork: tenderloin, bacon, kidneys

Veal: cutlet, shank, tenderloin, sweetbread, liver

Chicken and turkey: cutlet, skinless thigh, ham

Rabbit

Here are some examples of fatty meats:

Lamb: leg, ribs, brain

Beef: minced steak 10, 15, 20%, ribs, rib steak, tongue, marrow

Pork: ribs, brain, dry ham, black pudding, white pudding, bacon, terrine, rillettes, salami, sausage, sausages, and merguez

Veal: roast, paupiette, marrow, brain, tongue, dumplings

Chicken and turkey: thigh with skin

Guinea fowl

Capon

Turkey

Goose: foie gras

Lean or fatty fish

The fish does not contain carbohydrates so thatthat you can consume unlimited! As with meat, there are lean fish and fatty fish, pay attention to the amount of fat you eat and remember to vary your intake of fish. Oily fish have the advantage of containing a lot of good cholesterol, so it is beneficial for protection against cardiovascular disease! It will be advisable to consume fatty fish more than lean fish, to be able to manage your protein intake: if you consume lean fish, you will have a significant protein intake and little lipids, whereas with fatty fish, you will have a balanced protein and fat intake!

Here are some examples of lean fish:

> Cod
>
> Colin
>
> Sea bream
>
> Whiting
>
> Sole
>
> Turbot
>
> Limor career
>
> Location
>
> Pike
>
> Ray

Here are some examples of oily fish:

Swordfish

Salmon

Tuna

Trout

Monkfish

Herring

Mackerel

Cod

Sardine

Eggs

The eggs contain no carbohydrates, so you can consume as much as you want. It is often said that eggs are full of cholesterol and that you have to limit their intake, but the more cholesterol you eat, the less your body will produce by itself! In addition, it's not just poor-quality cholesterol so thatthat you can consume 6 per week without risk! And if you want to eat more but you are afraid for your cholesterol and I have not convinced you, remove the yellow!

Vegetables and raw vegetables

Yes, you can eat vegetables. But you have to be careful which ones: you can eat leafy vegetables (salad, spinach, kale, red cabbage, Chinese cabbage…) and flower vegetables (cauliflower, broccoli, Romanesco cabbage…) as well as avocado, cucumbers, zucchini or leeks, which do not contain many carbohydrates.

The oils

It's oil, so it's only fat, so it's unlimited to eat, but choose your oil wisely! Prefer olive oil, rapeseed, nuts, sunflower or sesame for example!

Foods authorized in moderate quantities.

The cold cuts

As you know, there is bad cholesterol in cold meats, so you will need to moderate your intake: eat it occasionally!

Fresh cheeses and plain yogurts

Consume with moderation because they contain carbohydrates.

Nuts and oilseeds

They have low levels of carbohydrates, but are rich in saturated fatty acids, that's why they should moderate their consumption. Choose almonds, hazelnuts, Brazil nuts or pecans.

Coconut (in oil, cream or milk)

It contains saturated fatty acids, that's why we limit its consumption. Cream and coconut oil contain a lot of medium chain triglycerides (MCTs), which increase the level of ketones, essential to stay in ketosis.

Berries and red fruits

They contain carbohydrates, in reasonable quantities, but you should not abuse them to avoid ketosis (blueberries, blackberries, raspberries...).

CHAPTER 3:

Over 250 Keto Recipes

Breakfast Recipes

1.   Almond flour keto pancakes

Preparation Time: 10 minutes

Cooking Time: 12 minutes

Servings: 10

Ingredients:

4 oz. softened cream cheese, at room temperature

Zest of 1 medium-sized lemon, fresh (approximately 1 teaspoon)

4 large-sized eggs, organic

½ cup almond flour

1 tablespoon butter, for frying and serving

Directions:

Combine the almond flour with eggs, cream cheese, and lemon zest using a whisk in a medium-sized mixing bowl until combined well, and completely smooth, for a minute or two.

The next step is to heat a large, nonstick skillet over medium heat until hot. Once done

add 1 tablespoon of butter until completely melted

swirl to coat the bottom completely.

Pour 3 tablespoons of the prepared batter (for each pancake) and cook for a minute or two, until turn golden. Carefully flip

cook the other side for 2 more minutes. Transfer to a clean, large plate and continue cooking with the remaining batter.

Top the cooked pancakes with some butter

serve immediately and enjoy.

Nutrition:

120 Calories 8.6g Total Fat

3.1g Saturated Fat 2g Total Carbohydrates

1g Dietary Fiber 0.8g Sugars

3.9g Protein

2.   Keto coconut flour egg muffin

Preparation Time: 5 minutes

Cooking Time: 10 minutes

Servings: 2

Ingredients:

1 organic egg, large-sized

2 teaspoons coconut flour or as required

A pinch of baking soda

1 tablespoon coconut oil, to coat

Salt, to taste

Directions:

Preheat your oven to 400°F. Lightly coat a large-sized coffee mug or ramekin dish with some coconut oil.

Using a fork

mix the entire ingredients together and make sure no lumps remain.

Bake for 10 to 12 minutes, until cooked through.

Cut in half

serve immediately and enjoy.

Nutrition:

48 Calories 3.9g Total Fat

1.1g Saturated Fat

1.7g Total Carbohydrates

0.3g Dietary Fiber

0.5g Sugars

3.7g Protein

3.   Broccoli   cheddar   cheese muffins

Preparation Time: 10 minutes

Cooking Time: 15 minutes

Servings: 6

Ingredients:

2/3 cup cheddar cheese, grated plus more for topping

¼ teaspoon garlic powder

¾ cup broccoli, steamed and chopped (fresh or frozen and thawed)

¼ teaspoon dried thyme

Directions:

Preheat your oven to 400°F. Combine the thyme with garlic powder in a large-sized mixing bowl until combined well and then, stir in the cheddar and broccoli. Evenly divide the mixture into the muffin tins (with 6 cups) filling each cup approximately 2/3 full.

Sprinkle with more of cheddar on top, if desired and then, bake until completely set, for 12 to 15 minutes. Serve immediately and enjoy.

Nutrition:

33 Calories

4.2g Total Fat

2.2g Saturated Fat

1.8g Total Carbohydrates

0.7g Dietary Fiber

0.3g Sugars

2.2g Protein

4. Chicken, bacon, avocado caesar salad

Preparation Time: 10 minutes

Cooking Time: 0 minutes

Servings: 4

Ingredients:

1 chicken breast, pre-cooked or grilled, sliced into small bite sized slices

1 avocado, ripe, sliced in half, twist and discard the pit, remove the shell and slice into approximately 1" slices.

Creamy Caesar dressing (approximately 3 tablespoons per salad)

1 cup bacon, pre-cooked, crumbled

Directions:

Combine the chicken breast with avocado slices and crumbled bacon between two large sized bowls.

Top with a few spoonfuls of the Creamy Caesar dressing

lightly toss the ingredients.

Serve immediately and enjoy.

Nutrition:

322 Calories

30g Total Fat

8.6g Saturated Fat

5g Total Carbohydrates

3.4g Dietary Fiber

0.9g Sugars

9.2g Protein

5. Coconut macadamia bars

Preparation Time: 15 minutes

Cooking Time: 0 minutes + refrigeration

Servings: 6

Ingredients:

½ cup macadamia nuts

6 tablespoons unsweetened coconut, shredded

½ cup almond butter

20 drops of stevia drops, preferably Sweetleaf

¼ cup coconut oil

Directions:

Crush the macadamia nuts using hands or in a food processor.

Combine coconut oil with the shredded coconut and almond butter in a large-sized mixing bowl. Add the stevia drops and chopped macadamia nuts.

Thoroughly mix and pour the prepared batter into a 9x9" baking dish lined with parchment paper.

Refrigerate for overnight

slice into desired pieces. Serve and enjoy.

Nutrition:

324 Calories 32g Total Fat

13g Saturated Fat

5g Total Carbohydrates

4g Dietary Fiber

1.8g Sugars

5.6g Protein

6. Macadamia chocolate fat bomb

Preparation Time: 15 minutes

Cooking Time: 0 + refrigeration

Servings: 6

Ingredients:

2 oz. cocoa butter

4 oz. macadamias, chopped

2 tablespoons Swerve

¼ cup coconut oil or heavy cream

2 tablespoons cocoa powder, unsweetened

Directions:

Fill a large sauce pan half full with boiling water. Place a small sized saucepan over the large sauce pan with the boiling water and melt the cocoa butter in it.

Once melted

add in the cocoa powder and then add the Swerve

mix well until the entire ingredients are completely melted and well blended.

Add in the macadamias

give everything a good stir.

Now, add the cream or coconut oil

mix well (bringing it to the temperature again). Pour the prepared mixture into paper candy cups or molds

filling them evenly. Let cool for a couple of minutes at room temperature and then place them in a refrigerator. Let chill until harden. Serve and enjoy.

Nutrition:

267 Calories

28g Total Fat

15g Saturated Fat

3g Total Carbohydrates

2g Dietary Fiber

0.9g Sugars

3g Protein

7. Keto lemon breakfast fat bombs

Preparation Time: 10 minutes

Cooking Time: 0 minutes + 50 minutes refrigeration

Servings: 6

Ingredients:

10 to 15 drops of Stevia extract

1 tablespoon lemon extract or lemon zest, organic

1 pack coconut butter or creamed coconut (approximately 3.5 oz.), softened

1 oz. extra virgin coconut oil, softened (approximately 1/8 cup)

A pinch of Himalayan pink salt or sea salt

Directions:

Zest the lemons and ensure that the coconut oil and coconut butter are at room temperature and softened.

Combine the entire ingredients together in a large-sized mixing bowl and ensure the stevia and lemon zest are evenly distributed.

Fill each silicone candy mold or mini muffin paper cup with approximately 1 tablespoon of the prepared coconut mixture and place them on a large-sized tray.

Place the tray inside the fridge and let chill until solid, for 40 to 50 minutes.

Keep refrigerated until ready to serve. Serve and enjoy.

Nutrition:

184 Calories

20g Total Fat

14g Saturated Fat

0.2g Total Carbohydrates

0.1g Dietary Fiber

0.1g Sugars

0.1g Protein

CHAPTER 4:

Lunch Recipes

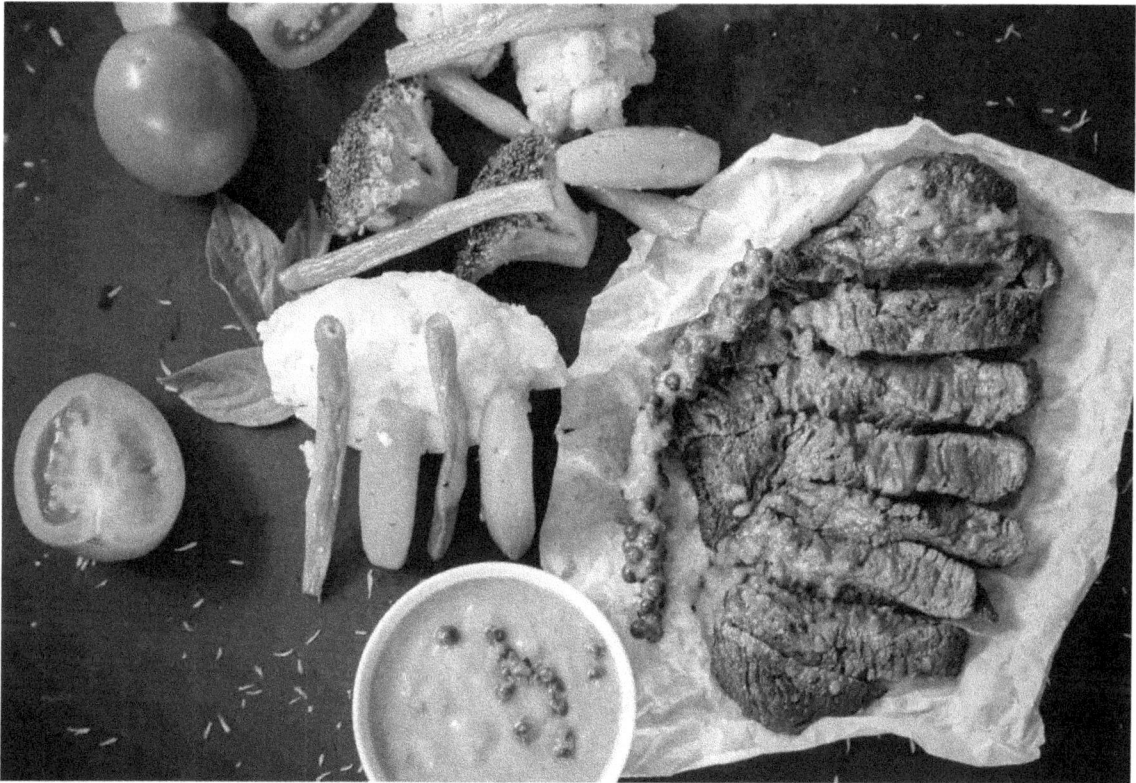

8. Cucumber Avocado Salad with Bacon

Preparation Time: 10 minutes

Cooking Time: None

Servings: 2

Ingredients:

2 cups fresh baby spinach, chopped

½ English cucumber, sliced thin

1 small avocado, pitted and chopped

1 ½ tablespoon olive oil

1 ½ tablespoon lemon juice

Salt and pepper

2 slices cooked bacon, chopped

Directions:

Combine the spinach, cucumber, and avocado in a salad bowl. Toss with olive oil, lemon juice, salt and pepper. Top with chopped bacon to serve.

Nutrition

Calories: 365 fat 24.5g

Protein: 7g Carbs: 13g Fiber: 8g

9. Bacon cheeseburger soup

Preparation Time: 10 minutes

Cooking Time: 15 minutes

Servings: 4

Ingredients:

4 slices uncooked bacon

8 ounces ground beef (80% lean)

1 medium yellow onion, chopped

1 clove garlic, minced

3 cups beef broth

2 tablespoons tomato paste

2 teaspoons Dijon mustard

Salt and pepper

1 cup shredded lettuce

½ cup shredded cheddar cheese

Directions:

Cook the bacon in a saucepan until crisp then drain on paper towels and chop.

Reheat the bacon fat in the saucepan and add the beef.

Cook until the beef is browned, then drain away half the fat.

Reheat the saucepan and add the onion and garlic – cook for 6 minutes.

Stir in the broth, tomato paste, and mustard then season with salt and pepper.

Add the beef and simmer on medium-low for 15 minutes, covered.

Spoon into bowls and top with shredded lettuce, cheddar cheese and bacon.

Nutrition

Calories: 315

fat 20g

Protein: 27g

Carbs: 6g

Fiber: 1g

10. Ham and Provolone Sandwich

Preparation Time: 30 minutes

Cooking Time: 5 minutes

Servings: 1

Ingredients:

1 large egg, separated

Pinch cream of tartar

Pinch salt

1-ounce cream cheese, softened

¼ cup shredded provolone cheese

3 ounces sliced ham

Directions:

For the bread, preheat the oven to 300°F and line a baking sheet with

parchment.

Beat the egg whites with the cream of tartar and salt until soft peaks form.

Whisk the cream cheese and egg yolk until smooth and pale yellow.

Fold in the egg whites a little at a time until smooth and well combined.

Spoon the batter onto the baking sheet into two even circles.

Bake for 25 minutes until firm and lightly browned.

Spread the butter on one side of each bread circle then place one in a preheated skillet over medium heat.

Sprinkle with cheese and add the sliced ham, then top with the other bread circle, butter-side-up.

Cook the sandwich for a minute or two then carefully flip it over.

Let it cook until the cheese is melted then serve.

Nutrition

Calories: 425g

fat 31g

Protein: 31g

Carbs: 5g

Fiber: 1g

11. Egg salad over lettuce

Preparation Time: 10 minutes

Cooking Time: None

Servings: 2

Ingredients:

3 large hardboiled eggs, cooled

1 small stalk celery, diced

3 tablespoons mayonnaise

1 tablespoon fresh chopped parsley

1 teaspoon fresh lemon juice

Salt and pepper

4 cups fresh chopped lettuce

Directions:

Peel and dice the eggs into a mixing bowl.

Stir in the celery, mayonnaise, parsley, lemon juice, salt and pepper.

Serve spooned over fresh chopped lettuce.

Nutrition:

Calories: 260

fat 23g

Protein: 10g

Carbs: 4g

Fiber: 1g

12. Egg drop soup

Preparation Time: 5 minutes

Cooking Time: 10 minutes

Servings: 4

Ingredients:

5 cups chicken broth

4 chicken bouillon cubes

1 ½ tablespoons chili garlic paste

6 large eggs, whisked

½ green onion, sliced

Directions:

Crush the bouillon cubes and stir into the broth in a saucepan.

Bring it to a boil, then stir in the chili garlic paste.

Cook until steaming, then remove from heat.

While whisking, drizzle in the beaten eggs.

Let sit for 2 minutes then serve with sliced green onion.

Nutrition:

Calories: 165

fat 9.5g

Protein: 16g

Carbs: 2.5g

Fiber: 0.5g

13. Bacon, lettuce, tomato, avocado sandwich

Preparation Time: 30 minutes

Cooking Time: None

Servings: 1

Ingredients:

1 large egg, separated

Pinch cream of tartar

Pinch salt

1 ounce cream cheese, softened

2 slices uncooked bacon

¼ cup sliced avocado

¼ cup shredded lettuce

1 slice tomato

Directions:

For the bread, preheat the oven to 300°F and line a baking sheet with parchment.

Beat the egg whites with the cream of tartar and salt until soft peaks form.

Whisk the cream cheese and egg yolk until smooth and pale yellow.

Fold in the egg whites a little at a time until smooth and well combined.

Spoon the batter onto the baking sheet into two even circles.

Bake for 25 minutes until firm and lightly browned.

Cook the bacon in a skillet until crisp, then drain on a paper towel.

Assemble the sandwich with the bacon, avocado, lettuce, and tomato.

Nutrition:

Calories: 335

fat 30g Protein: 16.5g

Carbs: 5.5g

Fiber: 2.5g

14. Spinach cauliflower soup

Preparation Time: 5 minutes

Cooking Time: 15 minutes

Servings: 4

Ingredients:

1 tablespoon coconut oil

1 small yellow onion, chopped

2 cloves garlic, minced

2 cups chopped cauliflower

8 ounces fresh baby spinach, chopped

3 cups vegetable broth

½ cup canned coconut milk

Salt and pepper

Directions:

Heat the oil in a saucepan over medium-high heat – add the onion and garlic.

Sauté for 4 to 5 minutes until browned, then stir in the cauliflower.

Cook for 5 minutes until browned, then stir in the spinach.

Let it cook for 2 minutes until wilted, then stir in the broth and bring to boil.

Remove from heat and puree the soup with an immersion blender.

Stir in the coconut milk and season with salt and pepper to taste. Serve hot.

Nutrition:

Calories: 165

fat 12g

Protein: 7g

Carbs: 9g

Fiber: 2.5g

15. Easy chopped salad

Preparation Time: 15 minutes

Cooking Time: None

Servings: 2

Ingredients:

4 cups fresh chopped lettuce

1 small avocado, pitted and chopped

½ cup cherry tomatoes, halved

¼ cup diced cucumber

2 hardboiled eggs, peeled and sliced

1 cup diced ham

½ cup shredded cheddar cheese

Directions:

Divide the lettuce between two salad plates or bowls.

Top the salads with diced avocado, tomato, and celery.

Add the sliced egg, diced ham, and shredded cheese.

Serve the salads with your favorite keto-friendly dressing.

Nutrition:

Calories: 520

fat 39.5g

Protein: 27g

Carbs: 17.5g

Fiber: 9g

16. Three Meat and Cheese Sandwich

Preparation Time: 30 minutes

Cooking Time: 5 minutes

Servings: 1

Ingredients:

1 large egg, separated

Pinch cream of tartar

Pinch salt

1-ounce cream cheese, softened

1-ounce sliced ham

1 ounce sliced hard salami

1-ounce sliced turkey

2 slices cheddar cheese

Directions:

For the bread, preheat the oven to 300°F and line a baking sheet with parchment.

Beat the egg whites with the cream of tartar and salt until soft peaks form.

Whisk the cream cheese and egg yolk until smooth and pale yellow.

Fold in the egg whites a little at a time until smooth and well combined.

Spoon the batter onto the baking sheet into two even circles.

Bake for 25 minutes until firm and lightly browned.

To complete the sandwich, layer the sliced meats and cheeses between the two bread circles.

Grease a skillet with cooking spray and heat over medium heat.

Add the sandwich and cook until browned underneath, then flip and cook until the cheese is melted.

Nutrition:

Calories: 610

fat 48g

Protein: 40g

Carbs: 3g

Fiber: 0.5g

17. Beef and Pepper Kebabs

Preparation Time: 30 minutes

Cooking Time: 10 minutes

Servings: 2

Ingredients:

2 tablespoons olive oil

1 ½ tablespoon balsamic vinegar

2 teaspoons Dijon mustard

Salt and pepper

8 ounces beef sirloin, cut into 2-inch pieces

1 small red pepper, cut into chunks

1 small green pepper, cut into chunks

Directions:

Whisk together the olive oil, balsamic vinegar, and mustard in a shallow dish.

Season the steak with salt and pepper, then toss in the marinade.

Let marinate for 30 minutes, then slide onto skewers with the peppers.

Preheat a grill pan to high heat and grease with cooking spray.

Cook the kebabs for 2 to 3 minutes on each side until the beef is done.

Nutrition:

Calories: 365

fat 21.5g

Protein: 35.5g

Carbs: 6.5g

Fiber: 1.5g

18. Slow-cooker chicken fajita soup

Preparation Time: 10 minutes

Cooking Time: 6 hours

Servings: 4

Ingredients:

12 ounces chicken thighs

1 cup diced tomatoes

2 cups chicken stock

½ cup enchilada sauce

2 ounces chopped green chiles

1 tablespoon minced garlic

1 medium yellow onion, chopped

1 small red pepper, chopped

1 jalapeno, seeded and minced

2 teaspoons chili powder

¾ teaspoon paprika

½ teaspoon ground cumin

Salt and pepper

1 small avocado, sliced thinly

¼ cup chopped cilantro

1 lime, cut into wedges

Directions:

Combine the chicken, tomatoes, chicken stock, enchilada sauce, chiles, and garlic in the slow cooker and stir well.

Add the onion, bell peppers, and jalapeno.

Stir in the seasonings, then cover and cook on low for 5 to 6 hours.

Remove the chicken and chop or shred then stir it back into the soup.

Spoon into bowls and serve with sliced avocado, cilantro, and lime wedges.

Nutrition:

Calories: 325 fat 17g

Protein: 28g Carbs: 17g Fiber: 7g

19. Avocado Egg Salad on Lettuce

Preparation Time: 10 minutes

Cooking Time: None

Servings: 2

Ingredients:

4 large hardboiled eggs, cooled and peeled

1 small avocado, pitted and chopped

1 medium stalk celery, diced

¼ cup diced red onion

2 tablespoons fresh lemon juice

Salt and pepper

4 cups chopped romaine lettuce

Directions:

Coarsely chop the eggs into a bowl.

Toss in the avocado, celery, red onion, and lemon juice.

Season with salt and pepper then serve over chopped lettuce.

Nutrition:

Calories: 375 fat 30g

Protein: 15.5g

Carbs: 15g

Fiber: 8g

20. Mediterranean keto dish

Preparation Time: 5 minutes

Cooking time: None

Servings: 2

Ingredients

1 Roma tomato, halved

1/4 cup olive oil

2 ounces fresh mozzarella cheese, sliced

2 ounces tuna, packed in water

8 green olives

Directions

Take two Serves plates and then distribute tomato, cheese, and tuna evenly between them.

Season with salt and black pepper and then serve with olive oil.

Nutrition:

Calories: 412

fat 35g

Protein: 20g

Carbs: 4g

Fiber: 1.5g

21. Spicy Zoodles with Cheese

Preparation Time: 10 minutes

Cooking time: 6 minutes

Servings: 2

Ingredients

1 ½ teaspoons minced garlic

1 large zucchini, spiralized into noodles

2 tablespoons grated parmesan cheese

2 tablespoons unsalted butter

Directions

Prepare zucchini noodles, and for this, cut zucchini into noodles by using a spiralizer or a vegetable peeler, and then set aside until required.

Bring out a skillet pan, place it over medium-high heat, add butter and garlic, cook for 1 minute until garlic is fragrant, then add zucchini noodles and continue cooking for 3 to 5 minutes until al dente.

When done, remove the skillet pan from heat, season zucchini noodles with salt, red chili flakes, and black pepper, add cheese, and stir well until mixed.

Nutrition:

Calories: 67.6

fat 7g

Protein: 3g

Carbs: 2.8g

Fiber: 0.5g

22. Spicy ground turkey dish

Preparation Time: 10 minutes

Cooking time: 27 minutes

Servings: 2

Ingredients

½ teaspoon minced garlic

¾ cup of water

1 jalapeno pepper, cored, cut into small cubes

4 ounces ground turkey

6 ounces tomato sauce

Directions

Bring out a skillet pan, place it over medium heat, add oil and when it melts, add turkey and cook for 3 to 4 minutes until turkey is slightly brown.

Then add garlic and jalapeno pepper, season with salt, red chili powder, cumin, and black pepper, stir well, and continue cooking for 3 minutes.

Add tomato sauce, water, stir well and simmer the chili for 20 to 25 minutes until the sauce has reduced and thickened to the desired level.

Taste the chili to adjust seasoning and serve with sliced avocado.

Nutrition:

Calories: 314

fat 20.1g

Protein: 24.1g

Net Carbs: 6.8g

Fiber: 4.1g

CHAPTER 5:

Dinner Recipes

23. Chicken Pan with Veggies and Pesto

Preparation Time: 10 minutes

Cooking time: 20 minutes

Servings: 4

Ingredients:

2 Tbsp olive oil

1-pound chicken thighs, boneless, skinless, sliced into strips

¾ cup oil-packed sun-dried tomatoes, chopped

1-pound asparagus ends

¼ cup basil pesto

1 cup cherry tomatoes, red and yellow, halved

Salt, to taste

Directions:

Heat olive oil in a frying pan over medium-high heat.

Put salt on the chicken slices and the put into a skillet, add the sun-dried tomatoes and fry for 5-10 minutes. Remove the chicken slices and season with salt. Add asparagus to the skillet. Cook for additional 5-10 minutes.

Place the chicken back in the skillet, pour in the pesto and whisk. Fry for 1-2 minutes.

Remove from the heat. Add the halved cherry tomatoes and pesto. Stir well and serve.

Nutrition:

Carbohydrates – 12 g

Fat – 32 g

Protein – 2 g

Calories – 423

24. Cabbage Soup with Beef

Preparation Time: 15 minutes

Cooking time: 20 minutes

Servings: 4

Ingredients:

2 Tbsp olive oil

1 medium onion, chopped

1-pound fillet steak, cut into pieces

½ stalk celery, chopped

1 carrot, peeled and diced

½ head small green cabbage, cut into pieces

2 cloves garlic, minced

4 cups beef broth

2 Tbsp fresh parsley, chopped

1 tsp dried thyme

1 tsp dried rosemary

1 tsp garlic powder

Salt and black pepper, to taste

Directions:

Heat oil in a pot (use medium heat). Add the beef and cook until it is browned. Put the onion into the pot and boil for 3-4 minutes.

Add the celery and carrot. Stir well and cook for about 3-4 minutes. Add the cabbage and boil until it starts softening. Add garlic and simmer for about 1 minute.

Pour the broth into the pot. Add the parsley and garlic powder. Mix thoroughly and reduce heat to medium-low.

Cook for 10-15 minutes.

Nutrition:

Carbohydrates – 4 g

Fat – 11 g

Protein – 12 g

Calories –177

25. Cauliflower Rice Soup with Chicken

Preparation Time: 10 minutes

Cooking time: 1 hour

Servings: 5

Ingredients:

2½ pounds chicken breasts, boneless and skinless

8 Tbsp butter

¼ cup celery, chopped

½ cup onion, chopped

4 cloves garlic, minced

2 12-ounce packages steamed cauliflower rice

1 Tbsp parsley, chopped

2 tsp poultry seasoning

½ cup carrot, grated

¾ tsp rosemary

1 tsp salt

¾ tsp pepper

4 ounces cream cheese

4¾ cup chicken broth

Directions:

Put shredded chicken breasts into a saucepan and pour in the chicken broth. Add salt and pepper. Cook for 1 hour.

In another pot, melt the butter. Add the onion, garlic, and celery. Saute until the mix is translucent. Add the riced cauliflower, rosemary, and carrot. Mix and cook for 7 minutes.

Add the chicken breasts and broth to the cauliflower mix. Put the lid on and simmer for 15 minutes.

Nutrition:

Carbohydrates – 6 g

Fat – 30 g

Protein – 27 g

Calories –415

26. Quick pumpkin soup

Preparation Time: 10 minutes

Cooking time: 20 minutes

Servings: 4-6

Ingredients:

1 cup coconut milk

2 cups chicken broth

6 cups baked pumpkin

1 tsp garlic powder

1 tsp ground cinnamon

1 tsp dried ginger

1 tsp nutmeg

1 tsp paprika

Salt and pepper, to taste

Sour cream or coconut yogurt, for topping

Pumpkin seeds, toasted, for topping

Directions:

Combine the coconut milk, broth, baked pumpkin, and spices in a soup pan (use medium heat). Stir occasionally and simmer for 15 minutes.

With an immersion blender, blend the soup mix for 1 minute.

Top with sour cream or coconut yogurt and pumpkin seeds.

Nutrition:

Carbohydrates – 8.1 g

Fat – 9.8 g Protein – 3.1 g

Calories – 123

27. Fresh avocado soup

Preparation Time: 5 minutes

Cooking time: 10 minutes

Servings: 2

Ingredients:

1 ripe avocado

2 romaine lettuce leaves, washed and chopped

1 cup coconut milk, chilled

1 Tbsp lime juice

20 fresh mint leaves

Salt, to taste

Directions:

Mix all your ingredients thoroughly in a blender .

Chill in the fridge for 5-10 minutes.

Nutrition:

Carbohydrates – 12 g

Fat – 26 g Protein – 4 g Calories – 280

28. Creamy garlic chicken

Preparation Time: 5 minutes

Cooking time: 15 minutes

Servings: 4

Ingredients:

4 chicken breasts, finely sliced

1 tsp garlic powder

1 tsp paprika

2 Tbsp butter

1 tsp salt

1 cup heavy cream

½ cup sun-dried tomatoes

2 cloves garlic, minced

1 cup spinach, chopped

Directions:

Blend the paprika, garlic powder, and salt and sprinkle over both sides of the chicken.

Melt the butter in a frying pan (choose medium heat). Add the chicken breast and fry for 5 minutes each side. Set aside.

Add the heavy cream, sun-dried tomatoes, and garlic to the pan and whisk well to combine. Cook for 2 minutes. Add spinach and saute for an additional 3 minutes. Return the chicken to the pan and cover with the sauce.

Nutrition:

Carbohydrates – 12 g

Fat – 26 g Protein – 4 g

Calories – 280

29.   Cauliflower cheesecake

Preparation Time: 20 minutes

Cooking time: 30 minutes

Servings: 6

Ingredients:

1 head cauliflower, cut into florets

⅔ cup sour cream

4 oz cream cheese, softened

1½ cup cheddar cheese, shredded

6 pieces bacon, cooked and chopped

1 tsp salt

½ tsp black pepper

¼ cup green onion, chopped

¼ tsp garlic powder

Directions:

Preheat the oven to 350°F.

Boil the cauliflower florets for 5 minutes.

In a separate bowl combine the cream cheese and sour cream. Mix well and add the cheddar cheese, bacon pieces, green onion, salt, pepper, and garlic powder. Put the cauliflower florets into the bowl and combine with the sauce.

Put the cauliflower mix on the baking tray and bake for 15-20 minutes.

Nutrition:

Carbohydrates – 8 g

Fat – 26 g Protein –15 g

Calories – 320

30.   Chinese pork bowl

Preparation Time: 5 minutes

Cooking time: 15 minutes

Servings: 4

Ingredients:

1¼ pounds pork belly, cut into bite-size pieces

2 Tbsp tamari soy sauce

1 Tbsp rice vinegar

2 cloves garlic, smashed

3 oz butter

1 pound Brussels sprouts, rinsed, trimmed, halved or quartered

½ leek, chopped

Salt and ground black pepper, to taste

Directions:

Fry the pork over medium-high heat until it is starting to turn golden brown.

Combine the garlic cloves, butter, and brussel sprouts. Add to the pan, whisk well and cook until the sprouts turn golden brown.

Stir the soy sauce and rice vinegar together and pour the sauce into the pan.

Sprinkle with salt and pepper.

Top with chopped leek.

Nutrition:

Carbohydrates – 7 g

Fat – 97 g

Protein – 19 g

Calories – 993

31. Turkey-pepper mix

Preparation Time: 20 minutes

Cooking time: 0 minutes

Servings: 1

Ingredients:

1 pound turkey tenderloin, cut in thin steaks

1 tsp salt, divided

2 Tbsp extra-virgin olive oil, divided

½ sweet onion, sliced

1 red bell pepper, cut into strips

1 yellow bell pepper, cut into strips

½ tsp Italian seasoning

¼ tsp ground black pepper

2 tsp red wine vinegar

1 14-ounces can crushed tomatoes, roasted

Fresh parsley

Basil

Directions:

Sprinkle ½ tsp salt on your turkey. Pour 1 Tbsp oil into the pan and heat it. Add the turkey steaks and cook for 1-3 minutes per side. Set aside.

Put the onion, bell peppers, and the remaining salt to the pan and cook for 7 minutes, stirring all the time. Sprinkle with Italian seasoning and add black pepper. Cook for 30 seconds. Add the tomatoes and vinegar and fry the mix for about 20 seconds.

Return the turkey to the pan and pour the sauce over it. Simmer for 2-3 minutes.

Top with chopped parsley and basil.

Nutrition:

Carbohydrates – 11 g

Fat – 8 g

Protein –30 g

Calories – 230

32.   Shrimp Scampi with Garlic

Preparation Time: 5 minutes

Cooking time: 10 minutes

Servings: 4

Ingredients:

1 pound shrimp

3 Tbsp olive oil

1 bulb shallot, sliced

4 cloves garlic, minced

½ cup Pinot Grigio

4 Tbsp salted butter

1 Tbsp lemon juice

½ tsp sea salt

¼ tsp black pepper

¼ tsp red pepper flakes

¼ cup parsley, chopped

Directions:

Pour the olive oil into the previously heated frying pan. Add the garlic and shallots and fry for about 2 minutes. Combine the Pinot Grigio, salted butter, and lemon juice. Pour this mix into the pan and cook for 5 minutes.

Put the parsley, black pepper, red pepper flakes, and sea salt into the pan and whisk well.

Add the shrimp and fry until they are pink (about 3 minutes).

Nutrition:

Carbohydrates – 7 g

Fat – 7 g Protein – 32 g

Calories – 344

33.   Simple tuna salad

Preparation Time: 5 minutes

Cooking time: 0 minutes

Servings: 4

Ingredients:

10 oz canned tuna, drained

1 avocado, chopped

1 rib celery, chopped

2 cloves fresh garlic, minced

3 Tbsp mayonnaise

1 red onion, chopped

Tbsp lemon juice

8 sprigs parsley

¼ cucumber, chopped

Salt and pepper, to taste

Directions:

Divide the parsley into two halves.

Mix all the ingredients except half of the parsley in a separate bowl. Stir well.

Add salt and pepper to taste.

Top with the remaining parsley.

Nutrition:

Carbohydrates – 1.7 g

Fat – 16.3 g Protein – 13.9 g

Calories – 225

Dinner is a very important meal for the day. Whether you are cooking for one or cooking for your whole family, dinner can truly bring people together. Hopefully, at this point in your day, you will be able to take some time to slow down and enjoy the process of cooking. If not, there are plenty of recipes that are still quick and easy to make the recipes to follow range for a variety of flavors for just about anyone.

34. Korma curry

Preparation Time: 10 minutes

Cooking time: 25 minutes

Servings: 6

Ingredients:

3-pound chicken breast, skinless, boneless

1 teaspoon of garam masala

1 teaspoon of curry powder

1 tablespoon of apple cider vinegar

½ cup of coconut cream

1 cup of organic almond milk

1 teaspoon of ground coriander

¾ teaspoon of ground cardamom

½ teaspoon of ginger powder

¼ teaspoon of cayenne pepper

¾ teaspoon of ground cinnamon

1 tomato, diced

1 teaspoon of avocado oil

½ cup of water

Directions:

Chop the chicken breast and put it in the saucepan.

Add avocado oil and start to cook it over the medium heat.

Sprinkle the chicken with garam masala, curry powder, apple cider vinegar, ground coriander, cardamom, ginger powder, cayenne pepper, ground cinnamon, and diced tomato. Mix up the ingredients carefully. Cook them for 10 minutes.

Add water, coconut cream, and almond milk. Saute the meat for 10 minutes more.

Nutrition: Calories 411

fat 19.3

fiber 0.9

carbs 6

protein 49.9

35. Zucchini bars

Preparation Time: 10 minutes

Cooking time: 15 minutes

Servings: 8

Ingredients:

3 zucchini, grated

½ white onion, diced

2 teaspoons of butter

3 eggs, whisked

4 tablespoons of coconut flour

1 teaspoon of salt

½ teaspoon of ground black pepper

5oz. of goat cheese, crumbled

4oz. of Swiss cheese, shredded

½ cup of spinach, chopped

1 teaspoon of baking powder

½ teaspoon of lemon juice

Directions:

In the mixing bowl, mix up together grated zucchini, diced onion, eggs, coconut flour, salt, ground black pepper, crumbled cheese, chopped spinach, baking powder, and lemon juice.

Add butter and churn the mixture until homogenous.

Line the baking dish with baking paper.

Transfer the zucchini mixture into the baking dish and flatten it.

Preheat the oven to 365F and put the dish inside. Cook it for 15 minutes. Then chill the meal well.

Cut it into bars.

Nutrition: Calories 199

fat 1316 fiber 215

carbs 7.1 protein 13.1

36.   Mushroom soup

Preparation Time: 10 minutes

Cooking time: 25 minutes

Servings: 4

Ingredients:

1 cup of water

1 cup of coconut milk

1 cup of white mushrooms, chopped

½ carrot, chopped

¼ white onion, diced

1 tablespoon of butter

2oz. turnip, chopped

1 teaspoon of dried dill

½ teaspoon of ground black pepper

¾ teaspoon of smoked paprika

1oz. of celery stalk, chopped

Directions:

Pour water and coconut milk in the saucepan. Bring the liquid to boil.

Add chopped mushrooms, carrot, and turnip. Close the lid and boil for 10 minutes.

Meanwhile, put butter in the skillet. Add diced onion. Sprinkle it with dill, ground black pepper, and smoked paprika. Roast the onion for 3 minutes.

Add the roasted onion in the soup mixture.

Then add chopped celery stalk. Close the lid.

Cook soup for 10 minutes.

Then ladle it into the serving bowls.

Nutrition: Calories 181

fat 17.3

fiber 2.5

carbs 6.9

protein 2.4

37. Stuffed portobello mushrooms

Preparation Time: 10 minutes

Cooking time: 10 minutes

Servings: 4

Ingredients:

2 portobello mushrooms

1 cup of spinach, chopped, steamed

2oz. of artichoke hearts, drained, chopped

1 tablespoon of coconut cream

1 tablespoon of cream cheese

1 teaspoon of minced garlic

1 tablespoon of fresh cilantro, chopped

3oz. of Cheddar cheese, grated

½ teaspoon of ground black pepper

2 tablespoons of olive oil

½ teaspoon of salt

Directions:

Sprinkle mushrooms with olive oil and place in the tray.

Transfer the tray in the preheated to 360F oven and broil them for 5 minutes.

Meanwhile, blend together artichoke hearts, coconut cream, cream cheese, minced garlic, and chopped cilantro.

Add grated cheese in the mixture and sprinkle with ground black pepper and salt.

Fill the broiled mushrooms with the cheese mixture and cook them for 5 minutes more. Serve the mushrooms only hot.

Nutrition:

Calories 183 fat 16.3

fiber 1.9 carbs 3 protein 7.7

38. Lettuce salad

Preparation Time: 10 minutes

Servings: 1

Ingredients:

1 cup of Romaine lettuce, roughly chopped

3oz. of seitan, chopped

1 tablespoon of avocado oil

1 teaspoon of sunflower seeds

1 teaspoon of lemon juice

1 egg, boiled, peeled

2oz. of Cheddar of cheese, shredded

Directions:

Place lettuce in the salad bowl. Add chopped seitan and shredded cheese.

Then chop the egg roughly and add in the salad bowl too.

Mix up together lemon juice with the avocado oil.

Sprinkle the salad with the oil mixture and sunflower seeds. Don't stir the salad before serving.

Nutrition:

calories 663 fat 29.5 fiber 4.7

carbs 3.8 protein 84.2

42 | P a g .

39. Onion soup

Preparation Time: 10 minutes

Cooking time: 25 minutes

Servings: 6

Ingredients:

2 cups of white onion, diced

4 tablespoon of butter

½ cup of white mushrooms, chopped

3 cups of water

1 cup of heavy cream

1 teaspoon of salt

1 teaspoon of chili flakes

1 teaspoon of garlic powder

Directions:

Put butter in the saucepan and melt it.

Add diced white onion, chili flakes, and garlic powder. Mix it up and saute for 10 minutes over the medium-low heat.

Then add water, heavy cream, and chopped mushrooms. Close the lid.

Cook the soup for 15 minutes more.

Then blend the soup until you get the creamy texture. Ladle it in the bowls.

Nutrition: calories 155

fat 15.1

fiber 0.9

carbs 4.7

protein 1.2

40. Asparagus salad

Preparation Time: 10 minutes

Cooking time: 15 minutes

Servings: 3

Ingredients:

10oz. of asparagus

1 tablespoon of olive oil

½ teaspoon of white pepper

4oz. of Feta cheese, crumbled

1 cup of lettuce, chopped

1 tablespoon of canola oil

1 teaspoon of apple cider vinegar

1 tomato, diced

Directions:

Preheat the oven to 365F.

Place asparagus in the tray, sprinkle with olive oil and white pepper, and transfer in the preheated oven. Cook it for 15 minutes.

Meanwhile, put crumbled Feta in the salad bowl.

Add chopped lettuce and diced tomato.

Sprinkle the ingredients with apple cider vinegar.

Chill the cooked asparagus to the room temperature and add in the salad.

Shake the salad gently before serving.

Nutrition:

calories 207 fat 17.6 fiber 2.4

carbs 6.8 protein 7.8

CHAPTER 6:

Vegetables Recipes

41. Keto spinach roll

Preparation Time: 10 minutes

Cooking time: 5 minutes

Servings: 15

Ingredients:

3 whole wheat tortillas

10-ounces spinach, frozen

½ cup sour cream

½ cup mayonnaise

Directions:

In a medium, pan cooks your spinach over medium heat and drain. Combine the sour cream, mayonnaise, and spinach in a mixing bowl. Spread the creamy mixture evenly over tortillas, roll them up and keep in fridge overnight. The next day cut into slices, serve and enjoy!

Nutrition:

Calories: 73

Cholesterol: 5 mg

Sugar: 0.6 g

Carbohydrates: 7.3 g

Protein: 1.7 g

fat 4.5 g

42. Artichoke avocado spinach salad

Preparation Time: 15 minutes

Cooking time: 0 minutes

Servings: 4

Ingredients:

4 cups spinach, fresh, washed

4 tablespoons lemon juice, fresh

1 avocado, peeled, diced

½ teaspoon garlic, minced

½ cup scallions, chopped

14-ounces artichoke hearts, drained, halved

¼ teaspoon pepper

1 teaspoon sugar or sugar substitute

Directions:

In a mixing bowl add artichokes, spinach, scallions, and avocado, toss well. In a small bowl mix together garlic, sugar, lemon juice and pepper. Pour mix over salad and serve fresh. Enjoy!

Nutrition: Calories: 168 fat 10.2 g

Cholesterol: 0 mg Sugar: 3 g

Carbohydrates: 18 g Protein: 5.4 g

43.   Corn lime avocado salad

Preparation Time: 15 minutes

Cooking time: 0 minutes

Servings: 6

Ingredients:

3 ears corn, cooked, cut kernels from cob

1 ripe avocado, peel, diced

1 garlic clove, minced

1 red bell pepper, cored, diced

1 jalapeno pepper, minced

1 scallion, sliced

Pepper to taste

1 tablespoon lime juice, fresh

2 tablespoons olive oil

Directions:

In a mixing bowl add scallion, garlic, corn, avocado, jalapeno, bell pepper and toss well. In a small bowl, combine lime juice with oil. Pour oil and juice mixture over salad and toss well. Season with pepper and serve fresh. Enjoy!

Nutrition:

Calories: 185

Sugar: 3.9 g

fat 12.2 g

Carbohydrates: 20 g

Cholesterol: 0 mg

Protein: 3.5 g

44.   Orange carrot kale salad

Preparation Time: 5 minutes

Cooking time: 12 minutes

Servings: 4

Ingredients:

8 cups kale, chopped

2 teaspoons olive oil

1 carrot, shredded

¼ teaspoon cumin, ground

1/8 teaspoon red chili flakes

1 onion, diced

2 garlic cloves, minced

1 red bell pepper, diced

1 cup fresh orange juice

1 teaspoon orange zest, grated

Pepper to taste

Directions:

In a pan over medium heat warm the olive oil. Add onion to the pan and sauté for 2 minutes. Add bell pepper, garlic, orange juice, kale and stir well. Reduce heat to medium-low and cook for another 5 minutes. Add in remaining ingredients and mix well. Cover and cook for an additional 5 minutes. Serve immediately and enjoy!

Nutrition:

Calories: 121 Carbohydrates: 23.3 g

fat 1.9 g Sugar: 5.2 g

Cholesterol: 0 mg

Protein: 5 g

45. Creamy Pumpkin Tomato Soup

Preparation Time: 10 minutes

Cooking time: 13 minutes

Servings: 4

Ingredients:

2 cups pumpkin, diced

½ teaspoon paprika

1 ½ teaspoons curry powder

½ cup onion, chopped

½ teaspoon garlic, minced

2 cups vegetable broth, low-sodium

1 teaspoon extra-virgin olive oil

½ cup tomato, chopped

Directions:

In a pan add the olive oil, onion, garlic and sauté over medium heat for 3 minutes. Add to pan remaining ingredients and bring to a boil. Reduce heat and cover, simmer for 10 minutes or until pumpkin is tender. Using blender puree the soup until smooth. Serve hot and enjoy!

Nutrition:

Calories: 84

Carbohydrates: 13.3 g

fat 2.4 g

Sugar: 5.6 g

Cholesterol: 0 mg

Protein: 4.3 g

46. Creamy Cauliflower Soup

Preparation Time: 10 minutes

Cooking time: 19 minutes

Servings: 4

Ingredients:

1 garlic clove, minced

½ head cauliflower, diced

1 small onion, diced

16-ounce vegetable broth

¼ tablespoon coconut oil

1 garlic clove, minced

½ teaspoon salt

Directions:

Heat the coconut oil in a pan over medium heat. Add onion, garlic and sauté for 4 minutes. Add vegetable broth and cauliflower. Bring to a boil. Cover and simmer for 15 minutes. Season with salt. Using blender puree the soup until smooth and creamy. Serve warm and enjoy!

Nutrition:

Calories: 53

Carbohydrates: 6.2 g

Sugar: 2.8 g

Cholesterol: 0 mg

fat 1.6 g

Protein: 4.1 g

47.   Spinach Garlic Salad

Preparation Time: 10 minutes

Cooking time: 2 minutes

Servings: 2

Ingredients:

1 garlic clove, minced

8-ounces spinach, fresh, washed

1 green onion, chopped

¼ teaspoon sea salt

1 ½ teaspoons extra-virgin olive oil

1 ½ teaspoons soy sauce

2 teaspoons sesame seeds, toasted

Directions:

Boil four cups of water in a pan over high heat. Once water is hot, blanch the spinach for 30 seconds. Remove the spinach from heat and rinse in cold water. Squeeze out excess water from spinach. In a bowl, add green onion, garlic, oil, sesame seeds, soy sauce, and salt. Add spinach and mix well. Serve fresh and enjoy!

Nutrition:

Calories: 80

Carbohydrates: 6.2 g

fat 5.4 g

Sugar: 0.8 g

Protein: 4.3 g

Cholesterol: 0 mg

48.   Almond peach arugula salad

Preparation Time: 15 minutes

Cooking time: 0 minutes

Servings: 4

Ingredients:

6 cups baby arugula, washed, dried

1 tablespoons water

¼ teaspoon pepper

½ cup almonds, toasted, sliced

3 ripe peaches, pitted and sliced

1 tablespoon balsamic vinegar

1 tablespoon olive oil

Pinch of salt

Directions:

In a mixing bowl, add arugula, almonds, and peaches. Toss well. In a small bowl, combine water, vinegar, salt and pour mixture over arugula mixture. Season with salt and pepper. Serve fresh and enjoy!

Nutrition:

Calories: 152

Carbohydrates: 14.3 g

fat 9.9 g

Sugar: 11.6 g

Cholesterol: 0 mg

Protein: 4.3 g

49.   Mushroom frittata

Preparation Time: 10 minutes

Cooking time: 46 minutes

Servings: 4

Ingredients:

6-ounces mushrooms, sliced

6 eggs, organic

1 cup leeks, sliced

Sea salt

Directions:

Preheat your oven to 350°Fahrenheit. Spray baking dish with cooking spray and set aside. Heat pan over medium heat. Spray pan with cooking spray. Add leeks and mushrooms to pan and sauté for 6 minutes. Break eggs in a bowl, whisk well. Transfer sautéed mushroom and leek mixture into prepared baking dish. Pour egg over mushroom mixture. Bake in preheated oven for 40 minutes. Serve warm and enjoy!

Nutrition:

Calories: 117

Cholesterol: 246 mg

Sugar: 2.1 g

fat 6.8 g

Carbohydrates: 5.1 g

Protein: 10 g

50.   Roasted Mushrooms

Preparation Time: 10 minutes

Cooking time: 30 minutes

Servings: 2

Ingredients:

2 tablespoons olive oil

10-ounces mushrooms, quartered

2 garlic cloves, sliced

1 teaspoon thyme, chopped

¼ teaspoon pepper

¼ teaspoon sea salt

Directions:

Preheat your oven to 400° Fahrenheit. Spray a baking tray with cooking spray and set aside. In a mixing bowl, combine mushrooms, thyme, oil, salt, and pepper. Spread mushrooms on prepared baking sheet and bake in preheated oven for 25 minutes. Add garlic and mix well and cook for an additional 5 minutes. Serve and enjoy!

Nutrition:

Calories: 157

Carbohydrates: 6.1 g

Sugar: 2.5 g

Cholesterol: 0 mg

fat 14.5 g

Protein: 4.7 g

51. Coconut almond egg wraps

Preparation Time: 10 minutes

Cooking time: 6 minutes

Servings: 4

Ingredients:

5 eggs, organic

2 tablespoons almond meal

1 tablespoon coconut flour

¼ teaspoon sea salt

Directions:

In your blender add all the ingredients and blend until smooth. Heat a pan over medium-high heat that is non-stick. Pour two tablespoons of batter into hot pan. Cover and cook for 3 minutes. Flip over and cook for an additional 3 minutes. Serve hot and enjoy!

Nutrition:

Calories: 111 fat 7.5 g

Carbohydrates: 3.1 g

Sugar: 0.8 g Cholesterol: 205 mg

Protein: 8.1 g

52. Baked egg tomato

Preparation Time: 5 minutes

Cooking time: 30 minutes

Servings: 2

Ingredients:

2 eggs, organic

2 large fresh tomatoes

1 teaspoon parsley, fresh, chopped

Pepper and salt to taste

Directions:

Preheat your oven to 350° Fahrenheit. Cut off the top of the tomato and spoon out the innards. Break an egg into each tomato, bake in preheated oven for 30 minutes. Season with parsley, pepper, and salt. Serve hot and enjoy!

Nutrition:

Calories: 96

fat 4.7 g

Carbohydrates: 7.5 g

Sugar: 5.1 g

Cholesterol: 164 mg

Protein: 7.2 g

53. Spicy asian style tofu

Preparation Time: 5 minutes

Cooking time: 15 minutes

Servings: 4

Ingredients:

14-ounces tofu, extra-firm, cut into cubes

1 tablespoon ginger, fresh, chopped

1 green Chili, chopped

1 tablespoon coconut oil

1 teaspoon apple cider vinegar

¼ teaspoon cayenne powder

2 garlic cloves, chopped

½ teaspoon basil, dried

2 teaspoon sesame seeds

1 teaspoon garlic salt

1 tablespoon soy sauce

1 teaspoon Worcestershire sauce

2 tablespoons Sriracha chili sauce

Pepper to taste

1 ½ tablespoons honey

Directions:

In a medium pan heat the coconut oil over medium heat. Add green chili, garlic and ginger, sauté for three minutes. Add tofu and sprinkle with some garlic salt. Sauté tofu until it is lightly golden brown for about 15 minutes. In a mixing bowl combine honey, cayenne powder, soy sauce, sriracha chili sauce, and Worcestershire sauce. Pour the honey mixture over the tofu and stir until well coated. Add basil leaves and sesame seeds and stir. Serve hot and enjoy!

Nutrition:

Calories: 154

fat 8.4 g

Cholesterol: 0 mg

Sugar: 9.6 g

Carbohydrates: 13.2 g

Protein: 9.1 g

54. Green Beans with Cheese

Preparation Time: 10 minutes

Cooking time: 5 minutes

Servings: 3

Ingredients:

1 lb. green beans

½ tablespoon butter

½ tablespoon coconut oil

1-ounce goat cheese

2 tablespoons walnuts, chopped

1 shallot, slices

Pepper and salt to taste

Directions:

Add salt and water in a pot and bring the water to a boil over medium heat. Add in the green beans and cook for 2 minutes, then drain and set aside. Heat the coconut oil in a pan over medium heat. Add the shallots and cook until softened. Add butter, once butter has melted add in the green beans and cook for an additional 3 minutes. Transfer beans into a bowl and toss with walnuts, cheese, pepper, and salt. Serve hot and enjoy!

Nutrition:

Calories: 168

fat 10.8 g

Carbohydrates: 13.8 g

Cholesterol: 15 mg

Sugar: 2.4 g

Protein: 7.2 g

55. Zucchini patties

Preparation Time: 10 minutes

Cooking time: 15 minutes

Servings: 6

Ingredients:

1 egg, organic, beaten

1 ½ cups zucchini, shredded

¼ cup breadcrumbs

¼ cup cheddar cheese, shredded

¼ teaspoon salt

1/8 teaspoon pepper

¼ teaspoon basil

¼ teaspoon garlic powder

Directions:

Preheat your oven to 425°Fahrenheit. Spray a baking tray with cooking spray and set aside. Place your shredded zucchini on a paper towel and pat it dry. Add zucchini and remaining ingredients into a mixing bowl and blend well. Drop a tablespoon of mixture on the prepared baking tray and lightly flatten with a spoon. Bake in preheated oven for 15 minutes or until golden brown. Serve warm and enjoy!

Nutrition:

Calories: 52 fat 2.6 g

Sugar: 0.9 g

Carbohydrates: 4.4 g

Cholesterol: 32 mg

Protein: 3.1 g

56. Cauliflower with artichokes pizza

Preparation Time: 10 minutes

Cooking time: 30 minutes

Serves 1

It is a delicacy that no one can resist. Suitable for vegetarians as it is a low-carb pizza. Filled with cheese and other delightful flavors, you will surely enjoy taking bites of the delicious crust.

ounces (120 g) grated cauliflower

2 ounces (57 g) canned artichokes, cut into wedges

ounces (120 g) shredded cheese

2 eggs, beaten

½ teaspoons salt

2 tablespoons tomato sauce

2 ounces (57 g) shredded cheese

2 ounces (57 g) mozzarella cheese

1 thinly sliced garlic clove

1 tablespoon dried oregano

Start by preheating the oven to 350°F (180°C).

In a bowl, add the cauliflower, shredded cheese, eggs and salt. Stir them properly.

Using a spatula, spread the mixture in a thin layer on a baking sheet lined with a parchment paper, approximately 11-inch (28 cm) in diameter.

Arrange the baking sheet in the oven and bake for 20 minutes or until they turn into a nice color.

Remove the baking sheet from your oven, spread with tomato sauce, then top with the cheese, garlic and artichokes. Sprinkle with oregano.

Increase the temperature of the oven to 420°F (215°C). Put the baking sheet back to the oven and bake the pizza for an extra 10 minutes.

Transfer the cooked pizza to a serving platter. Allow to cool for a few minutes before serving

STORAGE: Store in an airtight container in the fridge for up to 4 days or in the freezer for up to one month.

REHEAT: Microwave, covered, until the desired temperature is reached or reheat in a frying pan or air fryer / instant pot, covered, on medium.

SERVE IT WITH: To make this a complete meal, serve it with turmeric milkshake.

NUTRITION:

calories: 1010 total

fat 74g fiber: 7g

net carbs: 13g

protein: 68g

57.   Chili cabbage wedges

Preparation Time: 5 minutes

Cooking time: 20 minutes

Serves 4

This recipe calls for keto-friendly ingredients, including cabbage, olive oil and some spices. With minimal Preparation Time and simple cooking Directions, these chili cabbage wedges come together in a matter of minutes!

1 medium head cabbage

1 teaspoon chili powder

Pepper and salt

¼ cup olive oil

Start by preheating the oven to 400°F (205°C).

Divide the cabbage into wedges then spread them out on to a baking sheet.

Add the chili powder, pepper and salt to season. Sprinkle the olive oil on the cabbage and mix properly.

Put them in the oven. Bake for about 20 minutes or until the wedges turn to a nice color.

Transfer to four serving bowls. Allow to cool for a few minutes before serving.

STORAGE: Store in an airtight container in the fridge for up to 4 days or in the freezer for up to one month.

REHEAT: Microwave, covered, until the desired temperature is reached or reheat in a frying pan or air fryer / instant pot, covered, on medium.

SERVE IT WITH: To make this a complete meal, serve the wedges with tilapia fish.

NUTRITION:

calories: 108 total

fat 10g fiber: 3g

net carbs: 3g

protein: 1.5g

58. Cauliflower, leeks and broccoli

Preparation Time: 5 minutes

Cooking time: 15 minutes

Serves 4

You will enjoy the cheesy cauliflower that will incorporate the healthy broccoli. It is an easy-to-prepare recipe. This recipe is rich in nutrients with low carbohydrates. The inclusion of thyme makes the flavor wonderful.

8 ounces (227 g) cauliflower, chopped in bite-sized pieces

3 ounces (85 g) leeks, chopped in bite-sized pieces

1 pound (454 g) broccoli, chopped in bite-sized pieces

3 ounces (85 g) butter

5 ounces (142 g) shredded cheese

½ cup fresh thyme

4 tablespoons sour cream

Pepper and salt to taste

In a skillet over medium-high heat, add butter and heat to melt. Add the leeks, broccoli and cauliflower. Fry the vegetables until they become golden brown.

Add the cheese, thyme and sour cream. Stir well until the cheese melts. Add pepper and salt for seasoning.

Transfer them to a platter. Allow to cool for a few minutes before serving

STORAGE: Store in an airtight container in the fridge for up to 4 days or in the freezer for up to one month.

REHEAT: Microwave, covered, until the desired temperature is reached or reheat in a frying pan or air fryer / instant pot, covered, on medium.

SERVE IT WITH: To make this a complete meal, serve with mushroom pork chops.

NUTRITION:

calories: 368

total

fat 32g

fiber: 5.4g

net carbs: 9.3g

protein: 14.2g

59. Low-carb cheesy omelet

Preparation Time: 5 minutes

Cooking time: 10 minutes

Serves 2

This is a quick delicious meal that can be prepared quickly. One can take them as breakfast, lunch, or dinner. It is a satisfying meal that never disappoints. It is a glee to the taste buds.

6 eggs

7 ounces (198 g) shredded Cheddar cheese

Salt and ground black pepper, to taste

3 ounces (85 g) butter

In a bowl, whisk all the eggs until they are frothy and smooth. Add half of the Cheddar and blend well.

Add the pepper and salt to season.

In a frying pan, melt the butter over medium-high heat, then pour the egg mixture and cook for a few minutes until you see the eggs at the edges of the pan beginning to set.

Reduce the heat to low as you continue cooking the mixture for 3 minutes until it is almost cooked. Flip the omelet halfway through the cooking time. Scatter the remaining cheese on top and cook for another 1 to 2 minutes until the cheese melts.

Fold your omelet and serve while warm.

STORAGE: Store in an airtight container in the fridge for up to 4 days or in the freezer for up to one month.

REHEAT: Microwave, covered, until the desired temperature is reached or reheat in a frying pan or air fryer / instant pot, covered, on medium.

SERVE IT WITH: To make this a complete meal, serve the omelet with a tomato salad or avocado sticks.

NUTRITION:

calories: 899 total

fat 79g

fiber: 0g

net carbs: 5g

protein: 39.2g

60. Roasted green beans with parmesan

Preparation Time: 10 minutes

Cooking time: 20 minutes

Serves 4

An easy to prepare vegetable side dish that requires few ingredients. Can go with any protein. This meal can save you the hassle mostly when you have busy schedules. Try it out.

1 pound (454 g) fresh green beans

1 egg

½ teaspoon salt

¼ teaspoon pepper

2 tablespoons olive oil

1 teaspoon onion powder

1 ounce (28 g) grated Parmesan cheese

Start by preheating the oven to 400°F (205°C).

In a bowl, whisk the egg, salt, pepper, oil and the onion powder.

Add the green beans, then toss to coat well.

Drain the excess liquid, then arrange the green beans in a baking sheet lined with parchment paper. Sprinkle with Parmesan cheese.

Bake in the oven for about 20 minutes until the beans change to a nice color.

Transfer to four serving plates. Allow to cool for a few minutes before serving.

STORAGE: Store in an airtight container in the fridge for up to 4 days or in the freezer for up to one month.

REHEAT: Microwave, covered, until the desired temperature is reached or reheat in a frying pan or air fryer / instant pot, covered, on medium.

SERVE IT WITH: To make this a complete meal, serve it with roasted pork tenderloin or other food you like.

NUTRITION:

calories: 143 total

fat 11g

fiber: 2.5g

net carbs: 5.8g

protein: 6.2g

61. Roasted spicy brussels sprouts

Preparation Time: 5 minutes

Cooking time: 16 minutes

Serves 4

This is a low-carb side dish. It is a very delicious recipe. The mixture of the ingredients makes it rich in flavors. It is crispy and friendly to the whole family as it is not bitter at all.

1 pound (454 g) whole Brussels sprouts

2 tablespoons olive oil

1 onion, chopped

½ teaspoon ground black pepper

1 teaspoon salt

½ cup vegetable broth

Select the 'Sauté' function on your instant pot.

Coat the instant pot with the olive oil. Add the onions and cook for 2 minutes until they turn translucent.

Add the Brussels sprouts then cook them for an extra 1 minute.

Sprinkle with pepper and salt. Pour the vegetable broth over the Brussels sprouts. Close the lid of the instant pot.

Select the high-pressure function then set the timer to 3 minutes. Allow about 15 minutes for pressure to build-up.

Release the pressure using the quick-release procedure for about 5 minutes then unlock and take the lid off.

Transfer to four serving bowls. Allow to cool for a few minutes before serving.

STORAGE: Store in an airtight container in the fridge for up to 4 days or in the freezer for up to one month.

REHEAT: Microwave, covered, until the desired temperature is reached or reheat in a frying pan or air fryer / instant pot, covered, on medium.

SERVE IT WITH: To make this a complete meal, serve it with stewed beef steak.

NUTRITION:

calories: 123 total

fat 7.1g

carbs: 13.6g

protein: 4.3g

cholesterol: 0mg

sodium: 680mg

62. Spicy deviled eggs in curry paste

Preparation Time: 10 minutes

Cooking time: 10 minutes

Serves 6

This meal can be taken as an appetizer or a snack at any time. The curry adds the taste and flavor to the meal. An absolute easy to cook meal that takes minimum preparation time and Cooking time.

6 eggs

3 cups water

1 tablespoon red curry paste

½ cup keto-friendly mayonnaise

¼ teaspoon salt

½ tablespoon poppy seeds

In a pot of cold water. Boil the eggs for 7 minutes until well done. Reduce the heat to low and allow the eggs to simmer for 8 minutes. Cool them instantly in ice-cold water. Peel the eggs then divide the eggs into halves after cutting off both ends of the eggs.

Scoop the egg yolks out and place in a bowl.

Arrange the egg whites on a plate and place in the refrigerator. Mix the egg yolks, curry paste, and mayonnaise to form a smooth batter. Add salt to season. Remove egg whites from the refrigerator and top with the batter evenly.

Sprinkle the poppy seeds as toppings.

Transfer to six serving plates and serve.

STORAGE: Store in an airtight container in the fridge for up to 4 days or in the freezer for up to one month.

REHEAT: Microwave, covered, until the desired temperature is reached or reheat in a frying pan or air fryer / instant pot, covered, on medium.

SERVE IT WITH: To make this a complete meal, serve it with butter-fried green cabbage.

NUTRITION:

calories: 202 total

fat 20g fiber: 0g net carbs: 2g

protein: 6.2g

63. Chocolate sea salt smoothie

Preparation Time: 5 minutes

Cooking Time: 0 Minutes

Servings: 2

Ingredients:

1 avocado (frozen or not)

2 cups almond milk

1 tbsp tahini

¼ cup cocoa powder

1 scoop perfect Keto chocolate base

Directions:

Combine all the ingredients in a high speed blender and mix until you get a soft smoothie. Add ice and enjoy!

Nutrition:

Calories: 235 calories,

20g fat, 11.25 carbohydrates,

8g fiber, 5.5g protein

64. Eggplant lasagna

Preparation Time: 20 minutes

Cooking Time: 1 hour 10 minutes

Servings: 6

Ingredients:

1 Eggplant, large and sliced into thin rounds

1 TBSP Salt

1 C Marinara Sauce, low carb

.5 C Vegan Cheese, shredded

1 C Vegan Ricotta

Some Olive Oil

Directions:

Lay eggplant rounds in a single layer on a tray and liberally salt the slices, then flip them over and salt the other sides. Let stand for 1 hour so moisture beads up on the surface. Rinse the eggplant rounds and press them dry, as this will help you get out as much moisture as possible.

Turn your oven on to 350F. Brush a modest layer of olive oil over the bottom of an 8x8 baking dish, then make a single layer of eggplant rounds. Lightly layer marinara sauce over the eggplant layer, then top the layer with half of your vegan cheese shreds. Create another layer of eggplant rounds, then cover that layer with vegan ricotta and a thin layer of marinara sauce. Place one final layer of eggplant rounds on your lasagna, then spread the rest of your marinara sauce on the eggplant and the remaining vegan cheese on the sauce layer.

Bake your eggplant lasagna for 30 minutes, covered. Then, bake uncovered for an additional 15 minutes. Let it cool for 10 minutes before serving your eggplant lasagna.

Nutrition:

427kcal

65. Keto Vegan Cauliflower and Tofu Stir Fry

Preparation Time: 15 minutes

Cooking Time: 15 minutes

Servings: 4

Ingredients:

14 OZ Tofu, extra firm

TBSP Sesame Oil

1 Head Cauliflower, small cut into florets

2 Cloves Garlic, minced

.25 C Soy Sauce, low sodium

.5 TSP Chili Garlic Sauce

TBSP Peanut Butter, natural and salted

Directions:

Drain and press your tofu about 1.5 hours before you are ready to start preparing your stir fry so that it is completely dry when you start. When it is dry, cube it into 1" cubes. Turn your oven on to 400F. Cook tofu cubes for 25 minutes, then remove it from the oven and let your tofu cool down as you prepare the rest of your recipe. Whisk together sesame oil, soy sauce, chili garlic sauce, and peanut butter to prepare a marinade and let your tofu soak in it for 15 minutes so that it absorbs the flavor of the sauce. Place your cauliflower in a food processor or blender and pulse until it resembles cauliflower rice.

Heat excess marinade in a pan over the oven and then add the tofu and brown the edges of your tofu. Then, set them aside and heat your cauliflower rice in the excess sauce. The rice should cook for approximately 5-8 minutes, until it is slightly browned and tender.

Serve your tofu over your cauliflower rice right away using any leftover sauce, you may have to add even more flavor. Store leftovers in the fridge for up to 3 days, using a pan to reheat them when you are ready to eat more.

Nutrition:

Calories: 297 fat 15.6g,

Protein: 21.1g, Cholesterol 139.5mg

66.   Keto vegan curry

Preparation Time: 15 minutes

Cooking Time: 20 minutes

Servings: 4

Ingredients:

.25 C Vegan Butter

4 TBSP Coconut Oil, melted

16 OZ Tofu, extra firm and cubed

1 C Baby Spinach

1 Carrot, diced

1 Zucchini, diced

.5 Bell Pepper, sliced thin

2 Garlic Cloves, sliced thin

TBSP Vegan Red Curry Paste

1 C Vegetable Stock

C Coconut Milk, unsweetened and full fat

2 TBSP Peanut Butter, natural and unsweetened

2 TBSP Vegan Protein Powder, flavorless

4 Drops Liquid Stevia

.25 C Fresh Cilantro, chopped

1 TSP Salt

1 TSP Black Pepper

Directions:

Melt vegan butter over medium heat in a large stock pot. Add bell pepper and garlic and warm for about 1 minute, then add your curry paste. Stir constantly for 1 minute before adding your carrot, zucchini, coconut milk, protein powder, vegetable stock, stevia, peanut butter, and salt and pepper. Continue stirring until all ingredients are properly blended together.

Boil, then reduce your curry to a simmer and cook uncovered for about 8-10 minutes, until all of the vegetables are tender. Adjust your seasoning to your taste preferences.

Toss tofu cubes into the curry and simmer for an additional 5 minutes, so they are completely warmed all the way through, then add your spinach and cilantro, so they have time to wilt into the soup.

Serve coconut curry into four serving bowls and drizzle each bowl with 1 TBSP of the melted coconut oil.

Nutrition:

425 calories, 33g fat, 18g protein,

10g carbs, 2g sugars

67. Shirataki noodles with vegan alfredo sauce

Preparation Time: 10 minutes

Cooking Time: 15 minutes

Servings: 4

Ingredients:

1 Package Shirataki Noodles

1 Bag Cauliflower Rice

1 TBSP Lemon Juice

2 TBSP Avocado Oil

4 Cloves Garlic, minced

C Almond Milk, plain and unsweetened

C Cashews, soaked for at least 4 hours then drained

3 TBSP Nutritional Yeast

Directions:

Cook your shirataki noodles according to the Directions on the package.

Microwave cauliflower rice according to bag Directions, then remove to let the bag cool.

Warm avocado oil and minced garlic in a pan over medium heat until fragrant, then add the garlic mix, cauliflower rice, soaked cashews, almond milk, nutritional yeast, and lemon juice to a blender and blend it until smooth.

Pour your sauce back into the pan and add your cooked shirataki noodles and cook for about 7 minutes, until everything is warmed and well blended. Serve.

Nutrition:

340 calories

68. Cabbage hash browns

Preparation Time: 10 minutes

Cooking time: 12 minutes

Servings: 2

Ingredients

1 ½ cup shredded cabbage

2 slices of bacon

1/2 tsp garlic powder

1 egg

Seasoning:

1 tbsp coconut oil

½ tsp salt

1/8 tsp ground black pepper

Directions:

Crack the egg in a bowl, add garlic powder, black pepper, and salt, whisk well, then add cabbage, toss until well mixed and shape the mixture into four patties.

Take a large skillet pan, place it over medium heat, add oil and when hot, add patties in it and cook for 3 minutes per side until golden brown.

Transfer hash browns to a plate, then add bacon into the pan and cook for 5 minutes until crispy.

Serve hash browns with bacon.

Nutrition:

Calories: 336 Fats: 29.5 g

Protein: 16 g Net Carbohydrates: 0.9 g

Fiber: 0.8 g

69. Cauliflower hash browns

Preparation Time: 10 minutes

Cooking time: 18 minutes

Servings: 2

Ingredients

¾ cup grated cauliflower

2 slices of bacon

1/2 tsp garlic powder

1 large egg white

Seasoning:

1 tbsp coconut oil

½ tsp salt

1/8 tsp ground black pepper

Directions:

Place grated cauliflower in a heatproof bowl, cover with plastic wrap, poke some holes in it with a fork and then microwave for 3 minutes until tender.

Let steamed cauliflower cool for 10 minutes, then wrap in a cheesecloth and squeeze well to drain moisture as much as possible.

Crack the egg in a bowl, add garlic powder, black pepper, and salt, whisk well, then add cauliflower and toss until well mixed and sticky mixture comes together.

Take a large skillet pan, place it over medium heat, add oil and when hot, drop cauliflower mixture on it, press lightly to form hash brown patties, and cook for 3 to 4 minutes per side until browned.

Transfer hash browns to a plate, then add bacon into the pan and cook for 5 minutes until crispy.

Serve hash browns with bacon.

Nutrition:

Calories: 347.8

Fats: 31 g

Protein: 15.6 g

Net Carbohydrates: 1.2 g

Fiber: 0.5 g

70. Asparagus, With Bacon and Eggs

Preparation Time: 5 minutes

Cooking time: 12 minutes

Servings: 2

Ingredients:

4 oz asparagus

2 slices of bacon, diced

1 egg

Seasoning:

¼ tsp salt

1/8 tsp ground black pepper

Directions:

Take a skillet pan, place it over medium heat, add bacon, and cook for 4 minutes until crispy.

Transfer cooked bacon to a plate, then add asparagus into the pan and cook for 5 minutes until tender-crisp.

Crack the egg over the cooked asparagus, season with salt and black pepper, then switch heat to medium-low level and cook for 2 minutes until the egg white has set.

Chop the cooked bacon slices, sprinkle over egg and asparagus and serve.

Nutrition:

Calories: 179

Fats: 15.3 g

Protein: 9 g

Net Carbohydrates: 0.7 g

Fiber: 0.6 g

CHAPTER 7:

Poultry Recipes

71. Chicken avocado salad

Preparation Time: 10 minutes

Cooking Time: 10 minutes

Servings: 3

Ingredients:

2 chicken breasts, cooked and cubed

1 tbsp. fresh lime juice

2 avocados, peeled and pitted

2 Serrano chili peppers, chopped

1/4 cup celery, chopped

1 onion, chopped

1 cup cilantro, chopped

1 tsp kosher salt

Directions:

Scoop out avocados flesh using a spoon and place it into the bowl.

Mash the avocado flesh using a fork.

Add remaining ingredients & mix until well combined.

Serve and enjoy.

Nutrition:

Calories 236

Fat 10.6 g

Carbohydrates 4.5 g

Sugar 1 g Protein 29 g

Cholesterol 87 mg

72. Paprika chicken

Preparation Time: 10 minutes

Cooking Time: 35 minutes

Servings: 4

Ingredients:

4 chicken breasts, skinless & boneless, cut into chunks

2 tbsp. paprika

2 1/2 tbsp. olive oil

1 1/2 tsp garlic, minced

2 tbsp. fresh lemon juice

Pepper

Salt

Directions:

Preheat the oven to 350 F.

Now, in a small bowl, mix together garlic, lemon juice, paprika, and olive oil.

Season chicken with pepper and salt.

Spread 1/3 bowl mixture on the bottom of the casserole dish.

Add chicken into the casserole dish and rub with fish sauce.

Pour remaining sauce over chicken and rub well.

Bake for 30-35 minutes.

Serve and enjoy.

Nutrition:

Calories 380

Fat 22 g

Carbohydrates 2.6 g

Sugar 0.5 g

Protein 43 g

Cholesterol 130 mg

73. Parmesan chicken

Preparation Time: 10 minutes

Cooking Time: 35 minutes

Servings: 4

Ingredients:

1 lb. chicken breasts, skinless and boneless

1/2 cup parmesan cheese, grated

3/4 cup mayonnaise

1 tsp garlic powder

1/2 tsp Italian seasoning

Directions:

Preheat the oven to 375 F.

Spray baking dish with cooking spray.

Now, in a small bowl, mix together mayonnaise, garlic powder, poultry seasoning, and pepper.

Place chicken breasts into the prepared baking dish.

Spread mayonnaise mixture over chicken, then sprinkles cheese on top of chicken.

Bake chicken for 35 minutes.

Serve and enjoy.

Nutrition:

Calories 391

Fat 23 g

Carbohydrates 11 g

Sugar 3 g

Protein 33 g

Cholesterol 112 mg

74. Delicious chicken wings

Preparation Time: 10 minutes

Cooking Time: 30 minutes

Servings: 6

Ingredients:

1 egg, beaten

1 1/2 lbs. chicken wings

6 tbsp. olive oil

1/2 cup apple cider vinegar

1/2 tsp cayenne pepper

2 garlic cloves, minced

1/2 tsp pepper

3/4 tsp salt

Directions:

Add all ingredients except chicken in a large bowl and mix well.

Add chicken wings in a bowl and mix until well coated and set aside for 20 minutes.

Preheat the oven to 450 F.

Spray a baking tray with cooking spray.

Place marinated wings on a prepared baking tray and bake for 30 minutes. Serve and enjoy.

Nutrition:

Calories 355 Fat 23 g

Carbohydrates 0.5 g

Sugar 0.1 g Protein 33 g

Cholesterol 128 mg

75.   Lemon chicken

Preparation Time: 10 minutes

Cooking Time: 45 minutes

Servings: 8

Ingredients:

8 chicken breasts, skinless and boneless

1/4 cup fresh lemon juice

2 tbsp. green onion, chopped

1 tbsp. oregano leaves

3 oz. feta cheese, crumbled

1/4 tsp pepper

Directions:

Preheat the oven to 350 F.

Spray baking dish with cooking spray.

Place chicken breasts in prepared baking dish.

Drizzle with 2 tbsp. Lemon juice and sprinkle with 1/2 tablespoon oregano and pepper.

Top with green onion and crumbled cheese.

Drizzle with remaining lemon juice and oregano.

Bake for 45 minutes.

Serve and enjoy.

Nutrition:

Calories 246 Fat 10.8 g

Carbohydrates 1.2 g

Sugar 0.5 g Protein 34 g

Cholesterol 110 mg

76.   Yummy chicken skewers

Preparation Time: 10 minutes

Cooking Time: 10 minutes

Servings: 8

Ingredients:

2 lbs. chicken breast tenderloins

1 tsp lemon pepper seasoning

1 tsp garlic, minced

1 tbsp. olive oil

1 cup of salsa

Directions:

Add chicken in a zip-lock bag along with 1/4 cup salsa, lemon pepper seasoning, garlic, and oil.

Seal the bag and shake well and place it in the refrigerator overnight.

Thread marinated chicken onto the soaked wooden skewers.

And then, place skewers on hot grill and cooks for 8-10 minutes.

Brush with remaining salsa during the last 3 minutes of grilling.

Serve and enjoy.

Nutrition:

Calories 125

Fat 2.5 g

Carbohydrates 2.1 g

Sugar 1 g

Protein 24 g

Cholesterol 71 mg

77.   Tasty shredded chicken

Preparation Time: 10 minutes

Cooking Time: 25 minutes

Servings: 6

Ingredients:

3 chicken breast, boneless and skinless

1/4 cup vinegar

13.5 oz. chunky salsa

1/4 tsp onion powder

1 tbsp. ground cumin

1 1/2 tbsp. chili powder

Directions:

First, add all ingredients into the instant pot and stir well.

Seal pot with lid and cook on manual high pressure for 25 minutes.

Once done, then release pressure using the quick-release method than open the lid.

Remove chicken from pot and shred using a fork.

Serve and enjoy.

Nutrition:

Calories 171

Fat 6.3 g

Carbohydrates 5 g

Sugar 2.2 g

Protein 23 g

Cholesterol 64 mg

78.   Flavorful herb chicken

Preparation Time: 10 minutes

Cooking Time: 15 minutes

Servings: 5

Ingredients:

2 lbs. chicken breast, skinless and boneless

1/2 cup Greek yogurt

1/4 cup mayonnaise

1 1/2 tsp herb seasoning

1/2 tsp onion powder

1/2 tsp garlic powder

1/4 tsp salt

Directions:

Preheat the air-fryer to 380 F.

In a small bowl, mix together mayonnaise, herb seasoning, onion powder, garlic powder, and yogurt.

Coat chicken with mayo mixture.

Spray air-fryer basket with cooking spray.

Place chicken in an air-fryer basket and cook for 15 minutes. Turn halfway through.

Serve and enjoy.

Nutrition:

Calories 272 Fat 8 g

Carbohydrates 5 g

Sugar 2 g Protein 40 g

Cholesterol 121 mg

79.   Chicken bacon salad

Preparation Time: 10 minutes

Cooking Time: 10 minutes

Servings: 4

Ingredients:

2 chicken breasts, cooked and chopped

3 bacon slices, cooked and chopped

1/2 cup celery, diced

2 avocados, chopped

2 1/2 tbsp. olive oil

3 tbsp. fresh lemon juice

1/2 tsp dried dill

1 tbsp. dried chives

1/2 tsp pepper

1 tsp salt

Directions:

First, add all ingredients into the large bowl and toss well to combine.

Serve and enjoy.

Nutrition:

Calories 441

Fat 36 g

Carbohydrates 10 g

Sugar 1 g

Protein 24 g

Cholesterol 66 mg

80.   Easy crisp chicken wings

Preparation Time: 10 minutes

Cooking Time: 28 minutes

Servings: 3

Ingredients:

12 chicken wings

1/4 cup butter, melted

1/2 cup chicken stock

Pepper

Salt

Directions:

Pour chicken stock into the instant pot then place steamer rack in the pot.

Place chicken wings on top of the steamer rack.

Seal the pot with pressure cooking lid and cook on high pressure for 8 mins.

When done, release pressure using the quick-release method. Open the lid.

Remove chicken wings from instant pot and clean the pot.

Toss chicken wings with melted butter and season with pepper and salt.

Transfer chicken wings into the instant pot air fryer basket and place basket in the pot.

Seal pot with air fryer lid & select air fry mode then set the temperature to 400 F and timer for 10 minutes.

Mix chicken wings and air fry for 5-10 minutes more.

Serve and enjoy.

Nutrition:

Calories 784

Fat 47 g

Carbohydrates 2 g

Sugar 1 g

Protein 97 g

Cholesterol 343 mg

81. Sweet & savory orange chicken

Preparation Time: 10 minutes

Cooking Time: 14 minutes

Servings: 4

Ingredients:

4 chicken thighs

2 tbsp. honey

1/2 cup chicken stock

1 tbsp. wine

1 tbsp. olive oil

1 small onion, sliced

1 tbsp. ginger, minced

5 garlic cloves, chopped

1 orange juice

3 tbsp. water

2 1/2 tbsp. cornstarch

Salt

For marinade:

1/4 tsp sugar

1/2 tsp sesame oil

2 tbsp. soy sauce

1/4 tsp salt

Directions:

In a large bowl, mix together chicken, sugar, sesame oil, soy sauce, and salt and marinate for 30 minutes.

Then, add olive oil into the instant pot and set the pot on sauté mode.

Add ginger and onion and sauté for 2 minutes. Add garlic and sauté for 30 seconds.

Add wine and stir everything well. Add marinated chicken, orange juice, and stock and mix well.

Seal the pot with pressure cooking lid and cook on high pressure for 6 minutes. If done, allow releasing pressure naturally for 10 minutes then release the remaining pressure using quick release. Open the lid.

Remove chicken from pot & place on a plate. Then, in a small bowl, mix together cornstarch and 3 tbsp. Water & pour it into the instant pot.

Add honey and stir well and cook on sauté mode until sauce thickens. Pour sauce over chicken and coat well.

Clean the instant pot.

Place chicken in instant pot air fryer basket & place basket in the pot. Seal pot w/ air fryer lid and select broil mode and set timer for 5 minutes.

Serve and enjoy.

Nutrition:

Calories 400

Fat 11 g

Carbohydrates 23 g

Sugar 18 g

Protein 46 g

Cholesterol 130 mg

82. Lemongrass chicken

Preparation Time: 10 minutes

Cooking Time: 15 minutes

Servings: 4

Ingredients:

4 chicken thighs, bone-in

2 tbsp. brown sugar

3 tbsp. sugar

2 tbsp. fresh lime juice

3 tbsp. soy sauce

3 tbsp. fish sauce

1 tbsp. ginger, sliced

1 shallot, sliced

1 tbsp. garlic, chopped

2 lemongrass stalks, sliced

2 tbsp. water

1 1/2 tbsp. cornstarch

Directions:

In a mixing bowl, mix together chicken, 3 tbsp. Water, soy sauce, fish sauce, lime juice, brown sugar, lemongrass, ginger, shallot, and garlic. Cover & place in the refrigerator for 1 hour.

Place marinated chicken into the instant pot.

Seal pot with lid & cook on high pressure for 7 minutes.

When done, allow releasing pressure naturally for 10 mins. Then release the remaining pressure using quick release. Remove lid.

Remove chicken from pot and set aside.

Mix together cornstarch and 2 tbsp. Water and pour into the instant pot and cook on sauté mode until sauce thickens.

Pour sauce over chicken and coat well. Clean the instant pot.

Place chicken in instant pot air fryer basket and place basket in the pot.

Seal pot w/ air fryer lid & select broil mode & set timer for 5 minutes.

Serve and enjoy.

Nutrition:

Calories 374

Fat 19 g

Carbohydrates 25 g

Sugar 15 g

Protein 43 g

Cholesterol 130 mg

83. Juicy & tender whole chicken

Preparation Time: 10 minutes

Cooking Time: 25 minutes

Servings: 6

Ingredients:

3 lbs. whole chicken

1 tbsp. garlic, minced

3 tbsp. butter

8 cups of water

2 bay leaves

1 tsp dried thyme

1 tsp dried rosemary

1 tsp dried oregano

5 tsp sea salt

Directions:

Add water, thyme, rosemary, oregano, bay leaves, and salt into the instant pot and stir well.

Place chicken into the instant pot.

Seal the pot with pressure cooking lid and cook on high pressure for 0 minutes.

Once done, allow to release pressure naturally. Remove lid.

Remove chicken from pot and set aside. Clean the instant pot.

Then, melt butter in a pan over medium heat. Add garlic and sauté for 1 minute. Remove from heat.

Brush chicken with garlic butter.

Now, place the steamer rack in the instant pot, then places chicken on top of the rack.

Seal pot with air fryer lid and select broil mode and set timer for 5 minutes.

Serve and enjoy.

Nutrition:

Calories 486

Fat 27 g

Carbohydrates 1 g

Sugar 0 g

Protein 68 g

Cholesterol 217 mg

84. Chicken Breast with Vinegar Sauce

Servings: 4

Preparation Time: 10 minutes

Cooking Time: 35 Minutes

Ingredients:

2 Tbsp olive oil

2 lbs. of chicken breasts, boneless, cut into bite-size pieces

1 garlic clove, crushed

1/4 tsp ginger

3/4 tsp crushed red pepper flakes

1/4 cup white wine

2 Tbsp stevia granulated sweetener

1/3 cup coconut aminos (from coconut sap)

1 Tbsp apple cider vinegar (preferably non-pasteurized)

1/2 cup water

Directions:

Heat the olive oil in a large frying skillet.

Add the chicken pieces and cook until lightly browned.

Remove chicken, and place on a plate

set aside.

Add all remaining Ingredients in a skillet and stir for 3 - minutes over medium heat.

Add chicken, stir well, cover and simmer for 20 minutes over low heat.

Serve hot.

Nutrition:

Calories: 34

Carbohydrates: 2g

Proteins: 50g

Fat 13g

Fiber: 0.3g

85. Roasted turkey breast

Servings: 14

Preparation Time: 10 minutes

Cooking Time: 2½ Hours

Ingredients:

1 teaspoon onion powder

½ teaspoon garlic powder

Salt and ground black pepper, as required

1 (7-pound) bone-in turkey breast

1½ cups Italian dressing

Directions:

Preheat your oven to 325°F.

Grease a 13x9-inch baking dish.

In a bowl, add the onion powder, garlic powder, salt, and black pepper, and mix well.

Rub the turkey breast with the seasoning mixture generously.

Arrange the turkey breast into the prepared baking dish and top with the Italian dressing evenly.

Bake for about 2–2½ hours, coating with pan juices occasionally.

Remove from the oven and palace the turkey breast onto a platter for about 10–15 minutes before slicing.

With a sharp knife, cut the turkey breast into desired-sized slices and serve.

Nutrition:

Calories 45;Net Carbs 2.8 G ;

Total Fat 23.3 G ;Saturated Fat 5.2 G ;

Cholesterol 159 Mg ;Sodium 303 Mg ;

Total Carbs 2.8 G ;Fiber 0 G ;

Sugar 2.2 G ;Protein 48.7 G

86.   Stuffed chicken breasts

Servings: 4

Preparation Time: 10 minutes

Cooking Time: 30 Minutes

Ingredients:

1 teaspoon paprika

¼ teaspoon onion powder

¼ teaspoon garlic powder

Salt, to taste

4 grass-fed chicken breasts

1 tablespoon olive oil

4 ounces cream cheese, softened

¼ cup Parmesan cheese, grated

2 tablespoons mayonnaise

1½ cups fresh spinach, chopped

1 teaspoon garlic, minced

½ teaspoon red pepper flakes, crushed

Directions:

Preheat the oven to 375°F.

In a small bowl, mix together spices and salt.

Place the chicken breasts onto a cutting board and drizzle with oil.

Now, rub the chicken breasts with spice mixture evenly.

With a sharp knife, cut a pocket into the side of each chicken breast.

Place cream cheese, Parmesan, mayonnaise, spinach, garlic, red pepper, and ½ teaspoon of salt in a small mixing bowl and mix until well combined.

Stuff each chicken pocket with spinach mixture evenly.

Arrange the chicken breasts into a 9x13-inch baking dish.

Bake for about 25–30 minutes or until chicken is done completely.

Serve hot.

Nutrition:

Calories 468;Net Carbs 1.5 G;

Total Fat 30.2 G;

Saturated Fat G;Cholesterol 164 Mg;

Sodium 342 Mg;

Total Carbs 2.1 G;

Fiber 0.6 G Sugar 0.3 G;

Protein 45.7 G

87. Oven roasted creamy spiced chicken

Servings: 8

Preparation Time: 10 minutes

Cooking Time: 50 Minutes

Ingredients:

2 tsp of chicken fat

1 fresh whole chicken, cut up

1/2 cup ground almonds

1/4 tsp cayenne pepper

1/2 tsp onion powder

1/8 tsp ground ginger

1/2 tsp garlic powder

1/3 cup plain yogurt

Directions:

Preheat oven to 360°F/0°C.

Grease large baking tray with the chicken fat set aside.

Cut the chicken in large parts.

Rinse chicken pieces and pat dry.

In a large bowl, combine ground almonds, onion powder, garlic powder, cayenne pepper and ginger.

Dip chicken pieces in yogurt, and then roll in a ground almond mixture.

Place breaded chicken in prepared baking dish.

Bake, uncovered, for 45 to 50 minutes or until chicken is tender.

Nutrition:

Calories: 420

Carbohydrates 2.8g

Proteins 31g

Fat 321g

Fiber: 1g

88. Oven baked buffalo turkey wings

Servings: 6

Preparation Time: 10 minutes

Cooking Time: 1 Hour And 10 Minutes

Ingredients:

3 1/2 lbs. turkey wings, cut in half

3/4 cup almond flour

1/2 tsp salt to taste

1 tsp cayenne pepper

Olive oil for frying

1/4 cup almond butter melted

2 Tbsp of white vinegar

2 Tbsp hot red pepper sauce

2 Tbsp of fresh celery chopped

Directions:

Preheat the oven on 375°F/0°C.

Combine the almond flour, salt and cayenne pepper on a plate. Dust wings in almond flour mixture, shaking off excess.

Heat olive oil in a large heavy skillet over medium heat. Fry chicken for 10 minutes, turning once. Remove from heat and drain on kitchen paper towels.

Combine the almond butter, vinegar and hot pepper sauce in a small bowl. Place wings in a large baking pan

drizzle sauce over wings.

Bake wings for 1 hour, turning once halfway through.

Serve hot with fresh chopped celery.

Nutrition:

Calories: 549 Carbohydrates 2.5g

Proteins 63g Fat 31g Fiber: 1.2g

89.   Chicken breast stuffed with asparagus

Servings: 4

Preparation Time: 10 minutes

Cooking Time: 30 Minutes

Ingredients:

2 large skinless, boneless chicken breast halves

8 asparagus spears, trimmed

1/2 cup shredded parmesan cheese

1/4 cup ground almonds or Macadamia nuts

Salt and black pepper to taste

Directions:

Preheat oven to 375°F/0°C. Grease the baking dish

set aside.

Place each chicken breast between two sheets freezer bags on a solid surface.

Sprinkle each side with salt and pepper.

Place spears of asparagus down the center of a chicken breast and spread about 1/4 cup of parmesan cheese over the asparagus.

Repeat with the other chicken breast and roll the chicken around the asparagus and cheese to make a compact roll.

Place the rolls seam sides down in the prepared baking dish, and sprinkle each with about 2 tablespoons of ground almonds.

Bake for about 25 - 30 minutes.

Allow to cool for 10 minutes.

Serve warm.

Nutrition:

Calories: 236 Carbohydrates 3.8g

Proteins

Fat 32g Fiber: 2g

90.   Glazed chicken thighs

Servings: 8

Preparation Time: 10 minutes

Cooking Time: 35 Minutes

Ingredients:

½ cup balsamic vinegar

1/3 cup low-sodium soy sauce

3 tablespoons Yacon syrup

4 tablespoons olive oil

3 tablespoons chili sauce

2 tablespoons garlic, minced

Salt and ground black pepper, as required

8 (6-ounce) grass-fed skinless chicken thighs

Directions:

In a bowl, add all ingredients (except chicken thighs and sesame seeds) and beat until well combined.

In a large plastic zipper bag, add half of marinade and chicken thighs.

Seal the bag and shake to coat well.

Pace the bag in refrigerator for at least 1 hour, turning bag twice.

Reserve remaining marinade in the refrigerator until using.

Preheat your oven to 425°F.

In a small pan, add reserved marinade over medium heat and bring to a boil.

Cook for about 3–5 minutes, stirring occasionally.

Remove the pan of sauce from heat and set aside to cool slightly.

Remove the chicken from the bag and discard excess marinade.

Arrange chicken thighs into a 9x13-inch baking dish in a single layer and coat with some of the cooked marinade.

Bake for about 30 minutes, coating with the cooked marinade slightly after every 10 minutes.

Serve hot.

Nutrition:

Calories 406 ;

Net Carbs 4.4 G ;

Total Fat 19.6 G ;

Saturated Fat 4.5 G ;

Cholesterol 151 Mg ;

Sodium 880 Mg ;

Total Carbs 4.6 G ;

Fiber 0.1 G ;

Sugar 2.6 G ;

Protein 50 G

91. Broiled coconut aminos - glazed chicken drumsticks

Servings: 4

Preparation Time: 10 minutes

Cooking Time: 35 Minutes

Ingredients:

8 chicken drumsticks, skin-on or skinless

2 Tbsp of peanut butter

1/4 cup of coconut aminos (from coconut sap)

1/2 tsp ground ginger

1/2 tsp salt and freshly ground black pepper

Directions:

Preheat the oven's broiler, and line a broiler pan with aluminum foil.

In a large bowl, stir together peanut butter, coconut aminos, ginger, salt and pepper.

Add the chicken drumsticks and toss to coat. Refrigerate and marinate for one hour.

Remove the drumsticks from the fridge and place them in a prepared broiler pan.

Broil 13 to 1minutes, turn the drumsticks and broil for additional 5 minutes.

Serve hot.

Nutrition:

Calories: 351 Carbohydrates 2g

Proteins 55g Fat 13g Fiber: 0.6g

92. Slow cooked chicken salad with spinach

Servings: 4

Preparation Time: 10 minutes

Cooking Time: 5 Hours

Ingredients:

2 Tbsp of garlic-infused olive oil

1 1/2 lbs. chicken breast fillet

1 lbs. fresh spinach

1 red bell pepper cut into thin strips

1 red hot chili peppers (optional)

2 Tbsp mustard

1 Tbsp of fresh basil finely chopped

1 Tbsp of fresh mint finely chopped

1 tsp of coriander

Sea salt to taste

3 Tbs lemon juice (freshly squeezed)

Directions:

Pour the olive oil to the inner stainless-steel pot of Slow Cooker

place the spinach on the bottom.

Cut the chicken fillets into small cubes and place over spinach.

Add the bell pepper and red hot chili pepper (if used).

Combine all remaining Ingredients in a bowl and pour over chicken

gently stir with wooden spoon.

Cover and cook on LOW for 4-hours.

Adjust salt to taste and serve hot with lemon juice.

Nutrition:

Calories: 281 Carbohydrates 4.

Proteins 37.5g Fat 12g Fiber: 2g

93. Cold shredded chicken and cabbage salad

Servings: 4

Preparation Time: 10 minutes

Cooking Time: 30 Minutes

Ingredients:

1 lbs. red cabbage, shredded

2 cloves garlic, finely chopped

1 lbs. cooked chicken, shredded

4 Tbsp olive oil

3 Tbsp lemon juice (freshly squeezed)

Salt to taste

3 Tbsp mustard (Dijon, English, or whole grain)

Directions:

Shred the cabbage and place in a large salad bowl season with the salt and toss.

Add garlic over the cabbage. Add shredded chicken and pour with olive oil toss.

Add the mustard and gently stir with wooden spoon. Refrigerate for 30 minutes, sprinkle with the fresh lemon juice and serve.

Nutrition:

Calories: 209 Carbohydrates 7.3g

Proteins 23.5g Fat 9.5g Fiber: 3.3g

94.   Meatballs   in   mushroom sauce

Servings: 6

Preparation Time: 10 minutes

Cooking Time: 15 Minutes

Ingredients:

Meatballs

2 pounds ground turkey

2 medium eggs

1 onion, chopped finely

2 garlic cloves, minced

Salt and ground black pepper, to taste

Mushroom Sauce

1 tablespoon butter

3 ounces fresh mushrooms, chopped finely

3½ ounces cream cheese, softened

1 cup homemade chicken broth

Salt and ground black pepper, to taste

1 tablespoon fresh parsley, chopped

Directions:

Preheat the oven to 350°F. Line a baking sheet with a parchment paper.

For meatballs: Place all the ingredients into a large mixing bowl and with your hands, mix until well combined. Make golf ball-sized meatball from the mixture. Arrange the meatballs onto the prepared baking sheet in a single layer.

Bake for about 15 minutes, flipping once halfway through. For mushroom sauce: In a small saucepan, heat the oil over medium heat and cook the mushrooms for about 5–6 minutes.

Stir in the cream cheese and broth and cook for about 3–4 minutes, stirring frequently.

Stir in salt and black pepper and remove from the heat. Divide the meatballs onto serving plates and top with mushroom sauce. Garnish with parsley and serve.

Nutrition:

Calories 409; Net Carbs 2.7 G;

Total Fat 26.1 G;

Saturated Fat 8.1 G;

Cholesterol 232 Mg;

Sodium 401 Mg;

Total Carbs 3.3 G;

Fiber 0.6 G, Sugar 1.3 G;

Protein 46 G

95. Lemony chicken drumsticks

Servings: 6

Preparation Time: 10 minutes

Cooking Time: 40 Minutes

Ingredients:

3 pounds grass-fed chicken drumsticks

½ cup butter, melted

¼ cup fresh lemon juice

2 teaspoons garlic, minced

2 teaspoons Italian seasoning

Salt and ground white pepper, to taste

Directions:

Add butter, lemon juice, garlic, Italian seasoning, salt, and black pepper in a large mixing bowl and mix well.

Add the chicken drumsticks and coat with the marinade generously.

Cover the bowl and refrigerate for at least 5 hours.

Preheat the oven to 0°F.

Grease a large baking sheet.

Arrange the drumsticks onto the prepared baking sheet in a single layer.

Bake for approximately 40 minutes or until desired doneness.

Serve hot

Nutrition:

Calories 528;

Net Carbs 0.6 G;

Total Fat 28.8 G;

Saturated Fat 13.3 G;

Cholesterol 241 Mg;

Sodium 320 Mg;

Total Carbs 0.7 G;

Fiber 0.1 G

Sugar 0.4 G;

Protein 62.7 G

CHAPTER 8:

Meat Recipes

96.   Classic pork tenderloin

Preparation Time: 15 minutes

Cooking Time: 35 minutes

Servings: 4

Ingredients:

8 bacon slices

2 lb. pork tenderloin

1 tsp. dried oregano, crushed

1 tsp. dried basil, crushed

1 tbsp. garlic powder

1 tsp. seasoned salt

3 tbsp. butter

Directions:

Preheat the oven to 400 degrees F.

Heat a large ovenproof skillet over medium-high heat and cook the bacon for about 6-7 minutes.

Transfer the bacon onto a paper towel lined plate to drain.

Then, wrap the pork tenderloin with bacon slices and secure with toothpicks.

With a sharp knife, slice the tenderloin between each bacon slice to make a medallion.

In a bowl, mix together the dried herbs, garlic powder and seasoned salt.

Now, coat the medallion with herb mixture.

With a paper towel, wipe out the skillet.

In the same skillet, melt the butter over medium-high heat and cook the pork medallion for about 4 minutes per side.

Now, transfer the skillet into the oven.

Roast for about 17-20 minutes.

Remove the wok from oven and let it cool slightly before cutting.

Cut the tenderloin into desired size slices and serve.

Nutrition:

Calories: 471

Carbohydrates: 1g

Protein: 53.5g

fat 26.6g

Sugar: 0.1g

Sodium: 1100mg

Fiber: 0.2g

97. Signature italian pork dish

Preparation Time: 15 minutes

Cooking Time: 15 minutes

Servings: 6

Ingredients:

2 lb. pork tenderloins, cut into 1½-inch pieces

¼ C. almond flour

1 tsp. garlic salt

Freshly ground black pepper, to taste

2 tbsp. butter

½ C. homemade chicken broth

1/3 C. balsamic vinegar

1 tbsp. capers

2 tsp. fresh lemon zest, grated finely

Directions:

In a large bowl, add the pork pieces, flour, garlic salt and black pepper and toss to coat well.

Remove pork pieces from bowl and shake off excess flour mixture.

In a large skillet, melt the butter over medium-high heat and cook the pork pieces for about 2-3 minutes per side.

Add broth and vinegar and bring to a gentle boil.

Reduce the heat to medium and simmer for about 3-4 minutes.

With a slotted spoon, transfer the pork pieces onto a plate.

In the same skillet, add the capers and lemon zest and simmer for about 3-5 minutes or until desired thickness of sauce.

Pour sauce over pork pieces and serve.

Nutrition:

Calories: 373

Carbohydrates: 1.8g

Protein: 46.7g

fat 18.6g

Sugar: 0.4g

Sodium: 231mg

Fiber: 0.7g

98. Flavor packed pork loin

Preparation Time: 15 minutes

Cooking Time: 1 hour

Servings: 6

Ingredients:

1/3 C. low-sodium soy sauce

¼ C. fresh lemon juice

2 tsp. fresh lemon zest, grated

1 tbsp. fresh thyme, finely chopped

2 tbsp. fresh ginger, grated

2 garlic cloves, chopped finely

2 tbsp. Erythritol

Freshly ground black pepper, to taste

½ tsp. cayenne pepper

2 lb. boneless pork loin

Directions:

For pork marinade: in a large baking dish, add all the ingredients except pork loin and mix until well combined.

Add the pork loin and coat with the marinade generously.

Refrigerate for about 24 hours.

Preheat the oven to 400 degrees F.

Remove the pork loin from marinade and arrange into a baking dish.

Cover the baking dish and bake for about 1 hour.

Remove from the oven and place the pork loin onto a cutting board.

With a piece of foil, cover each loin for at least 10 minutes before slicing.

With a sharp knife, cut the pork loin into desired size slices and serve.

Nutrition:

Calories: 230 Carbohydrates: 3.2g

Protein: 40.8g fat 5.6g

Sugar: 1.2g Sodium: 871mg

Fiber: 0.6g

99.   Spiced pork tenderloin

Preparation Time: 15 minutes

Cooking Time: 18 minutes

Servings: 6

Ingredients:

2 tsp. fresh rosemary, minced

2 tsp. fennel seeds

2 tsp. coriander seeds

2 tsp. caraway seeds

1 tsp. cumin seeds

1 bay leaf

Salt and freshly ground black pepper, to taste

2 tbsp. fresh dill, chopped

2 (1-lb.) pork tenderloins, trimmed

Directions:

For spice rub: in a spice grinder, add the seeds and bay leaf and grind until finely powdered.

Add the salt and black pepper and mix.

In a small bowl, reserve 2 tbsp. of spice rub.

In another small bowl, mix together the remaining spice rub, and dill. Place 1 tenderloin over a piece of plastic wrap. With a sharp knife, slice through the meat to within ½-inch of the opposite side.

Now, open the tenderloin like a book.

Cover with another plastic wrap and with a meat pounder, gently pound into ½-inch thickness.

Repeat with the remaining tenderloin.

Remove the plastic wrap and spread half of the dill mixture over the center of each tenderloin.

Roll each tenderloin like a cylinder.

With a kitchen string, tightly tie each roll at several places.

Rub each roll with the reserved spice rub generously.

With 1 plastic wrap, wrap each roll and refrigerate for at least 4-6 hours.

Preheat the grill to medium-high heat. Grease the grill grate.

Remove the plastic wrap from tenderloins.

Place tenderloins onto the grill and cook for about 14-18 minutes, flipping occasionally.

Remove from the grill and place tenderloins onto a cutting board and with a piece of foil, cover each tenderloin for at least 5-10 minutes before slicing.

With a sharp knife, cut the tenderloins into desired size slices and serve.

Nutrition:

Calories: 313 Carbohydrates: 1.4g

Protein: 45.7g fat 12.6g

Sugar: 0g Sodium: 127mg Fiber: 0.7g

100. Sticky pork ribs

Preparation Time: 15 minutes

Cooking Time: 2 hours 34 minutes

Servings: 9

Ingredients:

¼ C. Erythritol

1 tbsp. garlic powder

1 tbsp. paprika

½ tsp. red chili powder

4 lb. pork ribs, membrane removed

Salt and freshly ground black pepper, to taste

1½ tsp. liquid smoke

1½ C. sugar-free BBQ sauce

Directions:

Preheat the oven to 300 degrees F. Line a large baking sheet with 2 layers of foil, shiny side out.

In a bowl, add the Erythritol, garlic powder, paprika and chili powder and mix well.

Season the ribs with salt and black pepper and then, coat with the liquid smoke.

Now, rub the ribs with the Erythritol mixture.

Arrange the ribs onto the prepared baking sheet, meaty side down.

Arrange 2 layers of foil on top of ribs and then, roll and crimp edges tightly.

Bake for about 2-2½ hours or until desired doneness.

Remove the baking sheet from oven and place the ribs onto a cutting board.

Now, set the oven to broiler.

With a sharp knife, cut the ribs into serving sized portions and evenly coat with the barbecue sauce.

Arrange the ribs onto a broiler pan, bony side up.

Broil for about 1-2 minutes per side.

Remove from the oven and serve hot.

Nutrition:

Calories: 530 Carbohydrates: 2.8g

Protein: 60.4g fat 40.3g Sugar: 0.4g

Sodium: 306mg Fiber: 0.5g

101.   Valentine's day dinner

Preparation Time: 15 minutes

Cooking Time: 35 minutes

Servings: 4

Ingredients:

1 tbsp. olive oil

4 large boneless rib pork chops

1 tsp. salt

1 C. cremini mushrooms, chopped roughly

3 tbsp. yellow onion, chopped finely

2 tbsp. fresh rosemary, chopped

1/3 C. homemade chicken broth

1 tbsp. Dijon mustard

1 tbsp. unsalted butter

2/3 C. heavy cream

2 tbsp. sour cream

Directions:

Heat the oil in a large skillet over medium heat and sear the chops with the salt for about 3-4 minutes or until browned completely.

With a slotted spoon, transfer the pork chops onto a plate and set aside.

In the same skillet, add the mushrooms, onion and rosemary and sauté for about 3 minutes.

Stir in the cooked chops, broth and bring to a boil.

Reduce the heat to low and cook, covered for about 20 minutes.

With a slotted spoon, transfer the pork chops onto a plate and set aside.

In the skillet, stir in the butter until melted.

Add the heavy cream and sour cream and stir until smooth.

Stir in the cooked pork chops and cook for about 2-3 minutes or until heated completely.

Serve hot.

Nutrition:

Calories: 400 Carbohydrates: 3.6g

Protein: 46.3g fat 21.6g

Sugar: 0.8g Sodium: 820mg

Fiber: 1.1g

102.   South east asian steak platter

Preparation Time: 15 minutes

Cooking Time: 20 minutes

Servings: 4

Ingredients:

14 oz. grass-fed sirloin steak, trimmed and cut into thin strips

Freshly ground black pepper, to taste

2 tbsp. olive oil, divided

1 small yellow onion, chopped

2 garlic cloves, minced

1 Serrano pepper, seeded and chopped finely

3 C. broccoli florets

3 tbsp. low-sodium soy sauce

2 tbsp. fresh lime juice

Directions:

Season steak with black pepper.

In a large skillet, heat 1 tbsp. of the oil over medium heat and cook the steak for about 6-8 minutes or until browned from all sides.

Transfer the steak onto a plate.

In the same skillet, heat the remaining oil and sauté onion for about 3-4 minutes.

Add the garlic and Serrano pepper and sauté for about 1 minute.

Add broccoli and stir fry for about 2-3 minutes.

Stir in cooked beef, soy sauce and lime juice and cook for about 3-4 minutes.

Serve hot.

Nutrition:

Calories: 282 Carbohydrates: 7.6g

Protein: 33.1g fat 13.5g

Sugar: 2.7g Sodium: 749mg Fiber: 2.3g

103. Pesto flavored steak

Preparation Time: 15 minutes

Cooking Time: 17 minutes

Servings: 4

Ingredients:

¼ C. fresh oregano, chopped

1½ tbsp. garlic, minced

1 tbsp. fresh lemon peel, grated

½ tsp. red pepper flakes, crushed

Salt and freshly ground black pepper, to taste

1 lb. (1-inch thick) grass-fed boneless beef top sirloin steak

1 C. pesto

¼ C. feta cheese, crumbled

Directions:

Preheat the gas grill to medium heat. Lightly, grease the grill grate.

In a bowl, add the oregano, garlic, lemon peel, red pepper flakes, salt and black pepper and mix well.

Rub the garlic mixture onto the steak evenly.

Place the steak onto the grill and cook, covered for about 12-17 minutes, flipping occasionally.

Remove from the grill and place the steak onto a cutting board for about 5 minutes.

With a sharp knife, cut the steak into desired sized slices.

Divide the steak slices and pesto onto serving plates and serve with the topping of the feta cheese.

Nutrition:

Calories: 226

Carbohydrates: 6.8g

Protein: 40.5g

fat 7.6g

Sugar: 0.7g

Sodium: 579mg

Fiber: 2.2g

104.   Flawless grilled steak

Servings: 5

Cooking Time: 10 minutes

Preparation Time: 21 minutes

Ingredients:

½ tsp. dried thyme, crushed

½ tsp. dried oregano, crushed

1 tsp. red chili powder

½ tsp. ground cumin

¼ tsp. garlic powder

Salt and freshly ground black pepper, to taste

1½ lb. grass-fed flank steak, trimmed

¼ C. Monterrey Jack cheese, crumbled

Directions:

In a large bowl, add the dried herbs and spices and mix well.

Add the steaks and rub with mixture generously.

Set aside for about 15-20 minutes.

Preheat the grill to medium heat. Grease the grill grate.

Place the steak onto the grill over medium coals and cook for about 17-21 minutes, flipping once halfway through.

Remove the steak from grill and place onto a cutting board for about 10 minutes before slicing.

With a sharp knife, cut the steak into desired sized slices.

Top with the cheese and serve.

Nutrition:

Calories: 271

Carbohydrates: 0.7g

Protein: 38.3g

fat 11.8g

Sugar: 0.1g

Sodium: 119mg

Fiber: 0.3g

CHAPTER 9:

Fish and Seafood Recipes

105. Keto fish

Preparation Time 40 minutes

Cooking Time: 30 minutes

Serving: 4

Ingredients:

For the Tartar Sauce

Four tablespoons dill pickle relish

1 cup mayonnaise

1/2 tablespoon curry powder

One tablespoon olive oil

1 1/2 pounds rutabaga (peeled and cleaned)

Salt and pepper, to taste

For the fish

1 1/2 pounds white fish

1 cup parmesan cheese (grated)

1 cup almond flour

Two eggs

2 cups coconut oil, for frying - One teaspoon paprika powder

1/4 teaspoon pepper - 1/2 teaspoon onion powder - One lemon

One teaspoon salt

Directions:

Take a small bowl and mix mayonnaise, curry powder, and pickle relish thoroughly. Refrigerate the tartar sauce until you finish the remaining dish.

Preheat the oven to 400 degrees Fahrenheit.

Slice the peeled rutabaga into thin rods and brush them with oil.

Line a baking tray with parchment paper and spread the oil-coated rutabaga rods.

Sprinkle the pepper and salt over the spread rutabaga.

Bake for 30 minutes until the rods become golden brown.

As the rutabaga gets cooked, Preparation, the fish.

Crack the eggs into a small bowl and beat it well with a fork.

Mix the Parmesan cheese, almond flour, paprika powder, pepper, onion powder, and salt on a plate. Set aside.

Dip the flour-coated fix into the beaten eggs and coat it again with the flour mix.

Pour the oil in a shallow skillet and heat over high heat.

If the rutabaga chips are ready by now, turn off the oven and let it sit for a while.

Fry the flour-egg coated fish in the hot oil until the fish is completely cooked and turns golden brown.

Repeat Directions 11 and 14 with the remaining fish.

Transfer the fried fish, baked rutabaga fries, and tartar into a serving bowl.

Serve hot and enjoy!

Nutrition:

Calories 463 Kcal

fat 26.2 g Protein: 49.2 g

Net carb: 4 g

106.   Zingy lemon fish
Preparation Time 50 minutes

Cooking Time: 40 minutes

Serving: 4

Ingredients:

14 ounces fresh Gurnard fish fillets

Two tablespoons lemon juice

Six tablespoons butter

½ cup fine almond flour

Two teaspoons dried chives

One teaspoon garlic powder

Two teaspoons dried dill

Two teaspoons onion powder

Salt and pepper to taste

Directions:

Add almond flour, dried herbs, salt, and spices on a large plate and stir until well combined. Spread it all over the plate evenly.

Place a large pan over medium-high heat. Add half the butter and half the lemon juice. When butter just melts, place fillets on the pan and cook for 3 minutes. Move the fillets around the pan so that it absorbs the butter and lemon juice.

Add remaining half butter and lemon juice. When butter melts, flip sides and cook the other side for 3 minutes.

Serve fillets with any butter remaining in the pan.

Nutrition:

Calories 406 Kcal

fat 30.33 g

Protein: 29 g - Net carb: 3.55 g

107.   Creamy keto fish casserole
Preparation Time 1 hour

Cooking Time: 50 minutes

Serving: 4

Ingredients:

25 ounces of white fish (slice into bite-sized pieces)

15 ounces broccoli (small florets, include the step too) - 3 ounces butter + extra

Six scallions (finely chopped) - 1 1/4 cups heavy whipping cream - Two tablespoons small capers

One tablespoon dried parsley - One tablespoon Dijon mustard

1/4 teaspoon black pepper (ground) - One teaspoon salt - Two tablespoons olive oil

5 ounces leafy greens (finely chopped), for garnishing

Directions:

Preheat the oven to 400 degrees Fahrenheit. Heat the oil in a saucepan over medium-high heat.

Fry the broccoli florets in the hot oil for 5 minutes until tender and golden.

Transfer the fried florets to a small bowl and season it with salt and pepper. Toss the contents to ensure all the florets get an equal amount of seasoning.

Add the chopped scallions and capers to the same saucepan and fry for 2 minutes. Return the florets to the pan and mix well.

Grease a baking tray with a little amount of butter and spread the fried veggies (broccoli, scallions, and capers) in the baking tray.

Add the sliced fish to the tray and nestle it among the veggies.

Mix the heavy cream, mustard, and parsley in a small bowl and pour this mixture over the fish-veggie mixture. Top this with the remaining butter and spread gently over the contents using a spatula. Transfer to a plate and garnish with chopped greens. Serve warm and enjoy!

Nutrition:

Calories 822 - Kcal

fat 69 g Protein: 41 g - Net carb: 8 g

108. Keto fish casserole with mushrooms and french mustard

Preparation Time 1 hour

Cooking Time: 50 minutes

Serving: 6

Ingredients:

25 ounces of white fish - 15 ounces mushrooms (cut into wedges)

20 ounces cauliflower (cut into florets) - 2 cups heavy whipping cream - 3 ounces butter

Two tablespoons Dijon mustard - 3 ounces olive oil - 8 ounces cheese (shredded)

Two tablespoons fresh parsley

Salt & pepper, to taste

Directions:

Preheat the oven to 350 degrees Fahrenheit

Fry the mushroom for 5 minutes until tender and soft.

Add the parsley, salt, and pepper to the mushrooms as you continue to mix well.

Reduce the heat and add the mustard and heavy whipping cream to the mushroom.

Allow it simmer for 10 minutes until the sauce thickens and reduces a bit.

Season the fish slices with pepper and salt. Set aside.

Sprinkle 3/4th of the cheese over the fish slices and spread the creamy mushroom over the top. Now again, top it with the remaining cheese.

Boil the cauliflower florets in lightly salted water for 5 minutes and strain the water.

Place the strained florets in a bowl and add the olive oil. Mash thoroughly with a fork until you get a coarse texture—season with salt and pepper. Mix well.

Nutrition:

Calories 828

fat 71 g

Protein: 39 g - Net carb: 8 g

109. Keto thai fish with curry and coconut

Preparation Time 50 minutes

Cooking Time: 40 minutes

Serving: 4

Ingredients:

25 ounces salmon (slice into bite-sized pieces)

15 ounces cauliflower (bite-sized florets)

14 ounces coconut cream

1-ounce olive oil

Four tablespoons butter

Salt and pepper, to taste

Directions:

Preheat the oven to 400 degrees Fahrenheit

Sprinkle salt and pepper over the salmon generously. Toss it once, if possible.

Place the butter generously over all the salmon pieces and set aside.

Pour this cream mixture over the fish in the baking tray.

Meanwhile, boil the cauliflower florets in salted water for 5 minutes, strain and mash the florets coarsely. Set aside.

Transfer the creamy fish to a plate and serve with mashed cauliflower. Enjoy!

Nutrition:

Calories 880 Kcal

fat 75 g

Protein: 42 g

Net carb: 6 g)

110. Keto salmon tandoori with cucumber sauce

Servings: 4

Ingredients

25 ounces salmon (bite-sized pieces) - Two tablespoons coconut oil

One tablespoon tandoori seasoning

For the cucumber sauce

1/2 shredded cucumber (squeeze out the water completely) - Juice of 1/2 lime

Two minced garlic cloves - 1 1/4 cups sour cream or mayonnaise

1/2 teaspoon salt (optional)

For the crispy salad

3 1/2 ounces lettuce (torn) - Three scallions (finely chopped)

Two avocados (cubed) - One yellow bell pepper (diced) - Juice of 1 lime

Directions:

Preheat the oven to 350 degrees Fahrenheit

Mix the tandoori seasoning with oil in a small bowl and coat the salmon pieces with this mixture.

Bake for 20 minutes until soft and the salmon flakes with a fork

Take another bowl and place the shredded cucumber in it. Add the mayonnaise, minced garlic, and salt (if the mayonnaise doesn't have salt) to the shredded cucumber.

Mix the lettuce, scallions, avocados, and bell pepper in another bowl. Drizzle the contents with the lime juice.

Transfer the veggie salad to a plate and place the baked salmon over it. Top the veggies and salmon with cucumber sauce.

Serve immediately and enjoy!

Nutrition:

Calories 847 Kcal fat 73 g

Protein: 35 g - Net carb: 6 g

111.   Creamy mackerel

This is creamy and rich!

Preparation time: 10 minutes

Cooking time: 20 minutes

Servings: 4

Ingredients:

Two shallots, minced

Two spring onions, chopped

Two tablespoons olive oil

Four mackerel fillets, skinless and cut into medium cubes

1 cup heavy cream

One teaspoon cumin, ground

½ teaspoon oregano, dried

A pinch of salt and black pepper

Two tablespoons chives, chopped

Directions:

Heat a pan with the oil over medium heat, add the spring onions and the shallots, stir and sauté for 5 minutes.

Add the fish and cook it for 4 minutes.

Add the rest of the ingredients, bring to a simmer, cook everything for 10 minutes more, divide between plates, and serve.

Nutrition:

Calories 403 Fat 33.9

Fiber 0.4 Carbs 2.7 Protein 22

112.   Lime mackerel

Preparation Time: 10 Minutes

Cooking Time: 30 Minutes

Servings: 4

Ingredients:

Four mackerel fillets, boneless

Two tablespoons lime juice

Two tablespoons olive oil

A pinch of salt and black pepper

½ teaspoon sweet paprika

Directions:

Arrange the mackerel on a baking sheet lined with parchment paper, add the oil and the other ingredients, rub gently, introduce in the oven at 360 degrees F and bake for 30 minutes.

Divide the fish between plates and serve.

Nutrition:

Calories 297

Fat 22.7

Fiber 0.2

Carbs 2

Protein 21.1

Directions:

Heat a pan with the oil over medium heat, add the spring onions and cook them for 2 minutes.

Add the fish, turmeric, and the other ingredients, cook for 5 minutes on each side, divide between plates and serve.

Nutrition:

Calories 205

Fat 8.6

Fiber 0.4

Carbs 1.1

Protein 31.8

113. Turmeric tilapia

Preparation time: 10 minutes

Cooking time: 12 minutes

Servings: 4

Ingredients:

Four tilapia fillets, boneless

Two tablespoons olive oil

One teaspoon turmeric powder

A pinch of salt and black pepper

Two spring onions, chopped

¼ teaspoon basil, dried

¼ teaspoon garlic powder

One tablespoon parsley, chopped

114. Walnut salmon mix

Preparation Time: 10 Minutes

Cooking Time: 14 Minutes

Servings: 4

Ingredients:

Four salmon fillets, boneless

Two tablespoons avocado oil

A pinch of salt and black pepper

One tablespoon lime juice

Two shallots, chopped

Two tablespoons walnuts, chopped

Two tablespoons parsley, chopped

Directions:

Heat a pan with the oil over medium-high heat, add the shallots, stir and sauté for 2 minutes.

Add the fish and the other ingredients, cook for 6 minutes on each side, divide between plates and serve.

Nutrition:

Calories 276

Fat 14.2

Fiber 0.7

Carbs 2.7

Protein 35.8

115.   Chives trout

Preparation Time: 10 Minutes

Cooking Time: 12 Minutes

Servings: 4

Ingredients:

Four trout fillets, boneless

Two shallots, chopped

A pinch of salt and black pepper

Three tablespoons chives, chopped

Two tablespoons avocado oil

Two teaspoons lime juice

Directions:

Heat a pan with the oil over medium heat, add the shallots and sauté them for 2 minutes.

Add the fish and the rest of the ingredients, cook for 5 minutes on each side, divide between plate sand serve.

Nutrition:

Calories 320

Fat 12

Fiber 1

Carbs 2

Protein 24

116.   Grilled mahi mahi

Preparation Time: 10 minutes

Cooking Time: 10 minutes

Servings: 6

Ingredients:

6 mahi-mahi fillets

¼ cup chicken stock ½ tsp garlic, minced

1 small onion, minced

6 tbsp butter

2 tbsp olive oil

2 tbsp lemon juice

Directions:

Preheat the grill to medium-high heat.

Place fish fillets during a bowl. Add oil, pepper, and salt over fish fillets and coat well.

Place fish on hot grill and cook for 3-4 minutes on all sides.

Transfer fish to a dish.

Melt 1 tbsp of butter during a pan over medium-high heat.

Add onion and sauté for two minutes or until onion is softened.

Add garlic and sauté for a moment.

Add stock and simmer until liquid is reduced by half.

Add juice and cook for a moment.

Remove pan from heat and add remaining butter and stir until sauce thickens.

Pour sauce over grilled fish and serve.

Nutrition:

Calories 237 Fat 16.2 g

Carbohydrates 1.2 g

Sugar 0.5 g Protein 21.3 g

Cholesterol 71 mg

117. Crab salad
Preparation Time: 10 minutes

Cooking Time: 10 minutes

Servings: 6

Ingredients:

8 oz crab meat

2 celery stalks, sliced

½ tsp Worcestershire sauce

½ tsp old bay spice

½ tsp dried dill

1 tsp lemon juice

2 tbsp fresh parsley, chopped

¼ cup mayonnaise

½ cup sour cream

4 oz cream cheese

1 tbsp garlic, crushed

¼ cup onion, diced

2 tbsp butter

Directions:

Melt butter during a small pan over medium heat.

Add onion and sauté until softened.

Add garlic and sauté for a moment.

Transfer onion-garlic mixture to the massive bowl. Add remaining ingredients to the bowl and stir everything well to mix. Serve and luxuriate in.

Nutrition:

Calories 219 Fat 18.4 g

Carbohydrates 5.6 g

Sugar 1.1 g Protein 7.2 g

Cholesterol 62 mg

118. Garlic shrimp
Preparation Time: 10 minutes

Cooking Time: 10 minutes

Servings: 4

Ingredients:

1 lb. shrimp

2 tbsp fresh parsley, chopped

½ cup parmesan cheese, grated

1 ½ cups heavy cream

½ cup chicken stock

5 garlic cloves, minced

2 tbsp butter

1 tbsp olive oil

Pepper Salt

Directions:

Heat vegetable oil during a large pan over medium-high heat.

Add shrimp to the pan and season with pepper and salt and cook shrimp for 1-2 minutes on all sides.

Transfer shrimp to the bowl and put aside.

Melt butter within the same pan. Add garlic and sauté for a moment.

Add stock and cook until the broth is reduced by half.

Turn heat to medium-low. Add cream and stir well and simmer for 2-3 minutes.

Add cheese and cook until cheese is melted.

Return shrimp to the pan.

Garnish with parsley and serve.

Nutrition:

Calories 453

Fat 32.4 g

Carbohydrates 4.5 g

Sugar 0.2 g

Protein 33.2 g

Cholesterol 331 mg

119. Easy seafood salad

Preparation Time: 10 minutes

Cooking Time: 3 minutes

Servings: 4

Ingredients:

8 oz shrimp

8 oz crab meat

1 tbsp dill, chopped

½ cup mayonnaise

2 tsp lemon juice

¼ tsp old bay seasoning

¼ cup onion, minced

½ cup celery, chopped

1 lemon, quartered

Pepper Salt

Directions:

Add lemon and water to the pot and convey to boil. Add shrimp to the pot and cook for 1-2 minutes. Drain shrimp well and place it during a large bowl.

Add remaining ingredients to the bowl and stir until well combined.

Cover salad bowl and place within the refrigerator for two hours.

Serve chilled and luxuriate in.

Nutrition:

Calories 240 Fat 11 g

Carbohydrates 10 g Sugar 2.4 g

Protein 20.6 g Cholesterol 157 mg

120.   Easy crab cakes

Preparation Time: 10 minutes

Cooking Time: 10 minutes

Servings: 2

Ingredients:

8 oz crab meat

2 tbsp butter

¼ tsp pepper

½ tsp old bay seasoning

2 tbsp mayonnaise

1 egg, lightly beaten

¼ cup almond flour

¼ cup red pepper, diced

1 small onion, diced

Directions:

Add all ingredients except butter during a bowl and blend until well combined.

Make small patties from bowl mixture. Melt butter during a pan over medium heat.

Fry crab cakes for 2-3 minutes on all sides or until lightly golden brown.

Serve and luxuriate in.

Nutrition:

Calories 311 Fat 20.7 g

Carbohydrates 10.3 g

Sugar 3.4 g

Protein 17.8 g

Cholesterol 177 mg

121.   Nutritious tuna patties

Preparation Time: 10 minutes

Cooking Time: 15 minutes

Servings: 8

Ingredients:

2 cans tuna, drained and flaked

4 tbsp olive oil

¼ cup fresh parsley, chopped

2 eggs, lightly beaten

3 garlic cloves, minced

2 tbsp Dijon mustard

2 tbsp mayonnaise

¼ tsp pepper

½ tsp salt

Directions:

Preheat the oven to 170 F.

In a bowl, mix tuna, parsley, eggs, garlic, Dijon mustard, mayonnaise, pepper, and salt.

Heat oil during a pan over medium heat.

Make small patties from tuna mixture and fry until golden brown, about 2-3 minutes per side.

Serve and luxuriate in.

Nutrition:

Calories 178 Fat 13.1 g

Carbohydrates 1.7 g

Sugar 0.4 g Protein 13.5 g

Cholesterol 56 mg

122. Quick butter cod

Preparation Time: 10 minutes

Cooking Time: 5 minutes

Servings: 4

Ingredients:

1 ½ lbs cod fillets, cut into pieces

½ tsp paprika

¼ tsp ground pepper

¼ tsp garlic powder

6 tbsp butter

½ tsp salt

Directions:

during a small bowl, mix paprika, pepper, garlic powder, and salt.

Coat fish pieces with seasoning mixture.

Melt 2 tbsp of butter during a large pan over medium-high heat.

Add fish pieces to the pan and cook for two minutes.

Turn heat to medium. Add remaining butter on top of fish pieces and cook for 3-4 minutes.

Once fish is cooked thoroughly, then remove the pan from heat. Add juice and stir well.

Serve and luxuriate in.

Nutrition:

Calories 291 Fat 18.8 g

Carbohydrates 0.4 g Sugar 0.1 g

Protein 30.6 g Cholesterol 129 mg

123. Baked tilapia

Preparation Time: 10 minutes

Cooking Time: 10 minutes

Servings: 4

Ingredients:

4 tilapia fillets

1 lemon zest

2 tbsp fresh lemon juice

1 tbsp garlic, minced

¼ cup butter, melted

2 tbsp fresh parsley, chopped

Pepper Salt

Directions:

Preheat the oven to 425 F.

during a small bowl, mix butter, lemon peel, juice, and garlic and put aside.

Season fish fillets with pepper and salt.

Place fish fillets onto the baking dish. Pour butter mixture over fish fillets.

Bake fish in a preheated oven for 10-12 minutes.

Garnish with parsley and serve.

Nutrition:

Calories 247 Fat 13.6 g

Carbohydrates 1 g

Sugar 0.2 g

Protein 32.4 g

Cholesterol 116 mg

124. Shrimp avocado salad

Preparation Time: 10 minutes

Cooking Time: 5 minutes

Servings: 4

Ingredients:

16 oz shrimp, thawed and drained

1 avocado, pitted and diced

¼ cup celery, chopped

1 small onion, chopped

2½ tbsp fresh dill, chopped

1 tbsp vinegar

1 tsp Dijon mustard

½ cup mayonnaise

Pepper Salt

Directions:

during a small bowl, mix mayonnaise, dill, vinegar, and mustard. Set aside.

Add shrimp, onion, and celery during a bowl.

Pour mayonnaise mixture over shrimp and stir well.

Cover and place within the refrigerator for 1-2 hours.

Add avocado and serve immediately.

Nutrition:

Calories 279 Fat 13.1 g

Carbohydrates 12.5 g

Sugar 2.7 g Protein 27 g

Cholesterol 246 mg

125. Paprika shrimp

Preparation Time: 10 minutes

Cooking Time: 50 minutes

Servings: 8

Ingredients:

2 lbs shrimp, peeled and deveined

1 tsp paprika

5 garlic cloves, sliced

3/4 cup olive oil

1/2 tsp red pepper flakes, crushed

1/4 tsp pepper

1 tsp kosher salt

Directions:

Add oil, red pepper flakes, pepper, paprika, garlic, and salt into the slow cooker and stir well.

Cover and cook on high for a half-hour.

Add shrimp. Stir and cook for 10 minutes.

Cover again and cook for 10 minutes more.

Serve and luxuriate in.

Nutrition:

Calories 300

Fat 20.2 g

Carbohydrates 2.7 g

Sugar 0.3 g

Protein 25 g

Cholesterol 240 mg

CHAPTER 10:

Cheeses

126. Smokey Cheddar Cheese (vegan)

Preparation Time: ~20 min

Cooking Time: 0 minutes

Servings: 8 / 1 block of cheese

Ingredients:

1 cup raw cashews (unsalted)

1 cup macadamia nuts (unsalted)

4 tsp. tapioca starch

1 cup water

¼ cup fresh lime juice

¼ cup tahini

½ tsp. liquid smoke

¼ cup paprika powder

½ tsp. ground mustard seeds

2 tbsp. onion powder

1 tsp. Himalayan salt

½ tsp. chili powder

1 tbsp. coconut oil

Directions:

Cover the cashews with water in a small bowl and let sit for 4 to 6 hours. Rinse and drain the cashews after soaking. Make sure no water is left.

Mix the tapioca starch with the cup of water in a small saucepan. Heat the pan over medium heat.

Bring the water with tapioca starch to a boil. After 1 minute, take the pan off the heat and set the mixture aside to cool down. Put all the remaining ingredients—except the coconut oil—in a blender or food processor. Blend until these ingredients are combined into a smooth mixture. Stir in the tapioca starch with water and blend again until all ingredients have fully incorporated. Grease a medium-sized bowl with the coconut oil to prevent the cheese from sticking to the edges. Gently pour the mixture into the bowl. Refrigerate the bowl, uncovered, for about 3 hours until the cheese is firm and ready to enjoy!

Alternatively, store the cheese in an airtight container in the fridge and consume within 6 days. Store for a maximum of 60 days in the freezer and thaw at room temperature.

Nutrition

Calories: 249 kcal Net Carbs: 6.9 g.

fat 21.7 g. Protein: 6.1 g.

Fiber: 4.3 g. Sugar: 2.6 g.

127.   Mozzarella Cheese (vegan)

Preparation Time: ~20 min

Cooking Time: 0 minutes

Servings: 16 / 1 block of cheese

Ingredients:

1 cup raw cashews (unsalted)

½ cup macadamia nuts (unsalted)

½ cup pine nuts

½ cup water

½ tbsp. coconut oil

½ tsp. light miso paste

2 tbsp. agar-agar

1 tsp. fresh lime juice

1 tsp. Himalayan salt

Directions:

Cover the cashews with water in a small bowl and let sit for 4 to 6 hours. Rinse and drain the cashews after soaking. Make sure no water is left.

Mix the agar-agar with the ½ cup of water in a small saucepan. Put the pan over medium heat.

Bring the agar-agar mixture to a boil. After 1 minute, take it off the heat and set the mixture aside to cool down.

Put all the other ingredients—except the coconut oil—in a blender or food processor. Blend until everything is well combined.

Add the agar-agar with water and blend again until all ingredients have been fully incorporated.

Grease a medium-sized bowl with the coconut oil to prevent the cheese from sticking to the edges. Gently transfer the cheese mixture into the bowl by using a spatula.

Refrigerate the bowl, uncovered, for about 3 hours until the cheese is firm

then serve and enjoy!

Alternatively, store the cheese in an airtight container in the fridge. Consume within 6 days. Store for a maximum of 60 days in the freezer and thaw at room temperature.

Nutrition

Calories: 101 kcal

Net Carbs: 2.1 g.

fat 9.2 g.

Protein: 2.2 g.

Fiber: 0.9 g.

Sugar: 0.9 g.

128.   Feta Cheese (vegan)

Preparation Time: ~20 min

Cooking Time: 0 minutes

Servings: 4

Ingredients:

1 13-oz. block extra firm tofu (drained)

3 cups water

¼ cup apple cider vinegar

2 tbsp. dark miso paste

1 tsp. ground black pepper

2 garlic cloves

1 tbsp. sun dried tomatoes (chopped)

2 tsp. Himalayan salt

Directions:

Cut the tofu into ½-inch cubes and put them into a medium-sized saucepan with 2 cups of water.

Bring the water to a boil over medium-high heat, take the pan off the heat immediately, drain half of the water, and set aside to let it cool down.

Pour the vinegar, miso paste, pepper, salt, and the remaining 1 cup of water into a blender or food processor. Blend until everything is well combined.

Pour the liquid from the blender into an airtight container. Add the garlic cloves, sundried tomatoes, and the tofu (including the water) to the container.

Give the feta cheese a good stir and then store in the fridge or freezer for at least 4 hours before serving.

Serve with low-carb crackers, or, enjoy this delicious feta cheese in a healthy salad!

Alternatively, store the cheese in an airtight container in the fridge and consume within 6 days. Store for a maximum of 30 days in the freezer and thaw at room temperature.

Nutrition

Calories: 101 kcal

Carbs: 5.2 g.

Net Carbs: 3.8 g.

fat 4.9 g.

Protein: 10.3 g.

Fiber:1.4 g.

Sugar: 0.7 g.

129.   Nut Free Nacho Dip (vegan)

Preparation Time: ~15 min

Cooking Time: 0 minutes

Servings: 8

Ingredients:

1 large eggplant (peeled and cubed)

2 medium Hass avocados (peeled, pitted, and halved)

¼ cup MCT oil

2 tsp. nutritional yeast

1 jalapeno pepper

1 red onion (diced)

1 garlic clove (halved)

¼ cup fresh cilantro (chopped)

1 tbsp. paprika powder

1 tsp. cumin seeds

1 tsp. dried oregano

½ tsp. Himalayan salt

Directions:

Slice the jalapeno in half lengthwise

remove the seeds, stem, and placenta, and discard.

Put the jalapeno and all other ingredients in a food processor or blender.

Mix everything into a smooth mixture. Use a spatula to scrape down the sides of the blender to make sure everything gets mixed evenly.

Transfer the dip to an airtight container.

Serve, share, and enjoy!

Alternatively, store the cheese in an airtight container in the fridge and consume within 2 days.

Tip: Serve with some celery sticks!

Nutrition

Calories: 135 kcal

Net Carbs: 3.5 g.

fat 12.3 g.

Protein: 1.8 g.

Fiber: 5.4 g.

Sugar: 2.7 g.

130. Black Olive & Thyme Cheese Spread (vegan)

Preparation Time: ~25 min

Cooking Time: 0 minutes

Servings: 16

Ingredients:

1 cup macadamia nuts (unsalted)

1 cup pine nuts

1 tsp. thyme (finely chopped)

1 tsp. rosemary (finely chopped)

2 tsp. nutritional yeast

1 tsp. Himalayan salt

10 black olives (pitted, finely chopped)

Directions:

Preheat the oven to 350°F / 175°C, and line a baking sheet with parchment paper.

Put the nuts on a baking sheet, and spread them out so they can roast evenly. Transfer the baking sheet to the oven and roast the nuts for about 8 minutes, until slightly browned.

Take the nuts out of the oven and set aside for about 4 minutes, allowing them to cool down.

Add all ingredients to a blender and process until everything combines into a smooth mixture. Use a spatula to scrape down the sides of the blender container in between blending to make sure everything gets mixed evenly.

Serve, share, and enjoy!

Alternatively, store the cheese in an airtight container in the fridge and consume within 6 days. Store for a maximum of 60 days in the freezer and thaw at room temperature.

Tip: Serve with some low-carb crackers!

Nutrition

Calories: 118 kcal

Net Carbs: 0.7 g.

fat 11.9 g.

Protein: 2 g.

Fiber: 1.4 g.

Sugar: 0.7 g.

131. Truffle Parmesan Cheese (vegan)

Preparation Time: ~30 min

Cooking Time: 0 minutes

Servings: 8

Ingredients:

1 cup macadamia nuts (unsalted)

1 cup raw cashews (unsalted)

2 garlic cloves

½ tbsp. nutritional yeast

2 tbsp. truffle oil

1 tsp. agar-agar

1 tsp. fresh lime juice

1 tsp. dark miso paste

Directions:

Cover the cashews with water in a small bowl and let sit for 4 to 6 hours. Rinse and drain the cashews after soaking. Make sure no water is left. Preheat the oven to 350°F / 175°C, and line a baking sheet with parchment paper.

Put the macadamia nuts on a baking sheet and spread them out, so they can roast evenly.

Transfer the baking sheet to the oven and roast the macadamia nuts for about 8 minutes, until slightly browned.

Take the nuts out of the oven and set them aside, allowing them to cool down.

Grease a medium-sized shallow baking dish with ½ tablespoon of truffle oil.

Add the soaked cashews, roasted macadamia nuts, and all the remaining ingredients to a blender or food processor. Blend everything into a crumbly mixture.

Transfer the crumbly parmesan into the baking dish, spread it out evenly, and firmly press it down until it has fused together into an even layer of cheese.

Cover the baking dish with aluminum foil and refrigerate the cheese for 8 hours or until the parmesan is firm.

Serve or store the cheese in an airtight container in the fridge and consume within 6 days. Store for a maximum of 60 days in the freezer and thaw at room temperature.

Nutrition

Calories: 202 kcal

Net Carbs: 4.4 g.

fat 18.7 g.

Protein: 4 g.

Fiber: 1.8 g.

Sugar: 1.8 g.

132. Gorgonzola 'Blue' Cheese (vegan)

Preparation Time: ~24 hours

Cooking Time: 0 minutes

Servings: 16

Ingredients:

½ cup macadamia nuts (unsalted)

½ cup pine nuts

1 cup raw cashews (unsalted)

1 capsule acidophilus (probiotic cheese culture)

½ tbsp. MCT oil

¼ cup unsweetened almond milk

1 tsp. ground black pepper

1 tsp. Himalayan salt

1 tsp. spirulina powder

Directions:

Cover the cashews with water in a small bowl and let sit for 4 to 6 hours. Rinse and drain the cashews after soaking. Make sure no water is left.

Preheat the oven to 350°F / 175°C, and line a baking sheet with parchment paper.

Spread the macadamia and pine nuts out on the baking sheet so they can roast evenly.

Put the baking sheet into the oven and roast the nuts for 8 minutes, until they are slightly browned.

Take the nuts out of the oven and allow them to cool down.

Grease a 3-inch cheese mold with the MCT oil and set it aside.

Add all ingredients—except the spirulina—to the blender or food processor. Blend on medium speed into a smooth mixture. Use a spatula to scrape down the sides of the blender to make sure all the ingredients get incorporated.

Transfer the cheese mixture into the greased cheese mold and sprinkle it with the spirulina powder. Use a small teaspoon to create blue marble veins on the cheese, and then cover the mold with parchment paper.

Place the cheese into a dehydrator and dehydrate the cheese at 90°F / 32°C for 24 hours.

Transfer the dehydrated cheese in the covered mold to the fridge. Allow the cheese to refrigerate for 12 hours.

Remove the cheese from the mold to serve in this condition, or, age the cheese in a wine cooler for up to 3 weeks. In case of aging the cheese, rub the outsides of the cheese with fresh sea salt. Refresh the salt every 2 days to prevent any mold. The cheese will develop a blue cheese-like taste, and by aging it, the cheese becomes even more delicious.

If the cheese is not aged, store it in airtight container and consume within 6 days.

Store the aged cheese in an airtight container and consume within 6 days, or for a maximum of 60 days in the freezer and thaw at room temperature.

Nutrition

Calories: 101 kcal

Net Carbs: 2 g.

fat 9.3 g.

Protein: 2.3 g.

Fiber: 1 g.

Sugar: 0.9 g.

CHAPTER 11:

Bagel Recipes

133. Vecheesy bagels

Preparation time: 45 minutes

Cooking Time: 0 minutes

Servings: 6

INGREDIENTS:

1 cup vegan cheese, shredded

6 tbsp aquafaba (the equivalent of 2 eggs)

1 cup coconut flour

2 tbsp bagel seasoning

Coconut oil, for greasing

DIRECTIONS:

Prepare the oven by heating it to 375 degrees F.

Use the coconut oil to grease the muffin tin.

Whip the aquafaba in a large bowl using a hand-held electric mixer for 6 minutes until it begins to form stiff peaks.

Combine the aquafaba, coconut flour, and both cheeses in a bowl and whisk together thoroughly.

Pour the batter into a muffin tin, sprinkle the seasoning over the top and bake for 20 minutes.

Once ready, remove from the oven and allow the bagels to cool down completely before serving.

Nutrition:

Calories: 218

fat 16g

Carbohydrates: 5g

Protein: 14g

Fiber: 1g

134. Garlic bagels

Preparation time: 15 minutes

Cooking Time: 0 minutes

Servings: 6

INGREDIENTS:

1/2 cup coconut flour

18 tbsp aquafaba (the equivalent of 6 eggs)

1 1/2 tsp garlic powder

1/3 cup coconut oil

1/2 tsp salt

1/2 tsp baking powder

DIRECTIONS:

Prepare the oven by heating it to 400 degrees F.

Use some of the coconut oil to grease the bagel tin and set it to one side

Whip the aquafaba in a large bowl using a hand-held electric mixer for 6 minutes until it begins to form stiff peaks.

Combine the aquafaba, coconut oil, garlic powder, and salt in a large bowl and whisk to combine.

Add the baking powder and the coconut flour and whisk to combine.

Pour the batter into the bagel tin and bake for 15 minutes.

Once ready, remove from the oven and allow the bagels to cool down completely before serving.

Nutrition:

Calories: 193 fat 15g

Carbohydrates: 4.6g Protein: 7.7g

Fiber: 3g

135. Cauliflower bagels

Preparation time: 45 minutes

Cooking Time: 0 minutes

Servings: 12

INGREDIENTS:

1 large cauliflower, roughly chopped

1/4 cup nutritional yeast

1/4 cup almond flour

1/2 tsp garlic powder

1 1/2 tsp salt

6 tbsp aquafaba (the equivalent of 2 eggs)

1 tbsp sesame seeds

DIRECTIONS:

Prepare the oven by heating it to 350 degrees F.

Use parchment paper to line a baking tray.

In a food processor, blend the cauliflower and then pour it into a bowl.

Add the garlic powder, almond flour, nutritional yeast, and salt. Stir to combine.

Whip the aquafaba in a large bowl using a hand-held electric mixer for 6 minutes until it begins to form stiff peaks.

Add the aquafaba to the cauliflower mixture. Stir to combine and then make bagels out of the dough.

Use your thumb to make a hole in the middle of each ball.

Arrange the bagels on the baking tray and flatten them out to make the shape of a bagel.

Sprinkle sesame seeds over the top and bake for 30 minutes.

Once ready, remove the bagels from the oven and allow them to cool down completely before serving.

Nutrition:

Calories: 53.1 fat 5.8g

Carbohydrates: 1.5g

Protein: 2g Fiber: 1.2g

136. Healthy bagels

Preparation time: 45 minutes

Cooking Time: 0 minutes

Servings: 6

INGREDIENTS:

1 cup coconut flour

1 tbsp baking powder

1/4 cup psyllium husk

1/2 cup hemp hearts

1/2 cup sesame seeds

1/2 cup pumpkin seeds

1 tsp salt

18 tbsp aquafaba (the equivalent of 6 eggs)

1 cup boiling water

DIRECTIONS:

Prepare the oven by heating it to 350 degrees F.

Use parchment paper to line a baking tray.

In a large bowl, combine the coconut flour, baking powder, psyllium husk, hemp hearts, sesame seeds, pumpkin seeds, and salt. Stir to combine.

Whip the aquafaba in a large bowl using a hand-held electric mixer for 6 minutes until it begins to form stiff peaks.

Combine the aquafaba with the coconut flour mixture and whisk to combine.

Add the water and continue to blend until the mixture forms into a smooth dough.

Form six balls out of the dough and use your thumb to make a hole in each ball.

Arrange the bagels on the baking tray and flatten them out a bit.

Once ready, remove the bagels from the oven and allow them to cool down completely before serving.

Nutrition:

fat 15.2g

Carbohydrates: 9.5g

Protein: 11.1g

Fiber: 2.3g

137. Raisin and cinnamon bagels

Preparation time: 45 minutes

Cooking Time: 0 minutes

Servings: 12

INGREDIENTS:

4 cups almond flour

115g raisins

1 cup lukewarm water

3 tbsp vegetable oil

2 tbsp ground cinnamon

4 tsp stevia

7g dried yeast

1 1/2 tsp salt

1/2 tsp baking soda

10-12 cups water

DIRECTIONS:

Combine the yeast, almond flour, stevia, baking soda, cinnamon, raisins, and salt in a large bowl.

Add the lukewarm water and stir to combine.

Add the oil and stir to combine.

Transfer the dough onto a lightly floured work surface and knead the dough for 10 minutes.

Coat the dough with oil and place it in a large bowl, cover it with a damp tea towel and leave it in a draft free area for 1 hour.

Once risen, split the dough into 12 and shape them into bagels.

Oil a baking sheet and arrange the bagels on it, cover with a damp tea cloth and leave to sit for 30 minutes.

In the meantime, preheat the oven to 390 degrees F.

Boil the water in a large saucepan.

Lightly oil two sheets of baking paper.

Reduce the temperature of the stove and place the bagels in the water for 90 seconds on each side.

Place kitchen towels on a plate, remove the bagels from the water and place them onto the kitchen towels to drain the water.

Arrange the bagels onto the baking tray.

Brush some oil over the bagels and bake for 15 minutes.

Once cooked, remove them from the oven and allow them to cool down before serving.

Nutrition:

Calories: 230

fat 6.4g

Carbohydrates: 4.3g

Protein: 2g

Fiber: 1.8g

138. New york bagels

Preparation time: 45 minutes

Cooking Time: 0 minutes

Servings: 8

INGREDIENTS:

FOR THE BAGELS:

3 1/3 cups almond flour

2 tbsp active dry yeast

1 1/2 cups warm water

1 1/2 tbsp stevia

1 1/2 tsp salt

10-12 cups water

FOR THE TOPPING:

Every bagel seasoning

1/4 cup almond milk

DIRECTIONS:

Combine the stevia with half a cup of warm water and then pour it onto the yeast. Stir gently and leave for 15 minutes.

In a large bowl, combine the salt and the almond flour.

Add the yeast mixture to the flour mixture and stir to combine and form a dough.

Flour a chopping board and knead the dough for 10 minutes.

Wet the dough and then place it inside a large bowl. Cover it with a damp tea towel and let it sit for 1 hour until the dough doubles in size.

Line a baking sheet with parchment paper and set it to one side.

Divide the dough into eight pieces and roll them out into balls.

Form a ring by poking out the center of the roll and arrange them on the baking sheet. Cover with a damp tea cloth and let it sit for 10 minutes .

Prepare the oven by heating it to 425 degrees F.

Boil a pot of water in a large saucepan over a high temperature.

Reduce the temperature to medium and then dip the bagels in the water and allow them to boil for two minutes on each side.

Place kitchen paper over a plate, take the bagels out of saucepan and drain them on the kitchen paper.

Arrange the bagels on the baking tray and brush them with the almond milk and then sprinkle the seasoning over the top.

Bake for bagels for 20 minutes, remove them from the oven and allow them to cool down for 10 minutes before serving.

Nutrition:

Calories: 226

fat 3.8g

Carbohydrates: 7g

Protein: 3g

Fiber: 1.1g

139.   Onion and herb bagels

Preparation time: 45 minutes

Cooking Time: 0 minutes

Servings: 8

INGREDIENTS:

4 cups almond flour

1 1/2 cups warm water

2 tbsp olive oil

2 tsp dried onion flakes

2 tsp salt

1 tbsp stevia

1 packet quick rise yeast

1/4 cup olive oil

1/4 tsp dried thyme

1/4 tsp dried sage

1/8 tsp garlic powder

10-12 cups water

DIRECTIONS:

In a large bowl, combine the warm water, salt and stevia, stir to combine and then sprinkle the yeast over the top. Allow the yeast mixture to sit for five minutes until it starts to foam.

Add the almond flour and olive oil and whisk to combine.

Use your hands to knead the dough for five minutes.

Add the thyme, sage, onion, and garlic powder and continue to knead until everything is combined.

Cover the dough with olive oil and then cover it with cling film and leave it to sit in a draft free area for one hour until the dough rises to double its size.

Place the dough on a lightly floured chopping board and cut the dough into eight pieces.

Roll the dough out into logs and then join the ends to form a bagel.

Lay parchment paper over a baking tray and arrange the bagels on the tray. Cover them with a damp kitchen towel and leave them to rise for 20 minutes.

In the meantime, prepare the oven by heating it to 425 degrees F.

Boil the water in a large saucepan over high temperature and dip the bagels in the water for 30 seconds.

Remove the bagels from the water and arrange them on the baking tray.

Brush the bagels with olive oil and bake them for 20 minutes.

Once cooked, remove the bagels from the oven and leave them to cool for 10 minutes before serving.

Nutrition:

Calories: 386

fat 9.7g

Carbohydrates: 6.2g

Protein: 3g

Fiber: 4g

CHAPTER 12:

Soup Recipes

140. Broccoli cheese soup

Preparation Time: 10 minutes

Cooking Time: 30 minutes

Servings: 4

Ingredients:

2 garlic cloves, minced

½ cup heavy cream

1 ½ cups bone or chicken or vegetable broth

2 cups broccoli, cut into florets

1 ½ cups cheddar cheese, shredded

Directions:

Over medium heat in a large pot sauté the garlic until fragrant, for a minute.

Add the chicken broth, chopped broccoli and heavy cream. Increase the heat and bring everything together to a boil. Once boiling decrease the heat and let simmer until the broccoli is tender, for 10 to 20 minutes.

Slowly add in the shredded cheddar cheese and continue to cook until melted, stirring constantly, over very low heat settings (if required, work in batches and don't cook over high heat). Once the cheese melts completely immediately remove the pot from heat. Serve warm and enjoy.

Nutrition:

471 Calories

38g Total Fat

19g Saturated Fat

5.7g Total Carbohydrates

1.2g Dietary Fiber

1.8g Sugars

26g Protein

141. Cauliflower, Leek, and Bacon Soup

Preparation Time: 5 minutes

Cooking Time: 55 minutes

Servings: 4

Ingredients:

4 cups vegetable or chicken broth

½ head of cauliflower

cut into small pieces

8 bacon slices

1 leek

cut into small pieces

Pepper and salt to taste

Directions:

Place the leek and cauliflower pieces into a large pot and then fill the pot with chicken broth.

Bring it to a boil over moderate heat settings until tender, for 30 to 35 minutes.

To create a smooth soup

puree the vegetables using an immersion blender.

Microwave the bacon slices on high-heat settings for a minute and then cut into small pieces

dropping the pieces into the soup.

Cook for 20 more minutes on low-heat.

Add pepper and salt to taste.

Nutrition:

122 Calories

6.6g Total Fat

2g Saturated Fat

5.5g Total Carbohydrates

2.8g Dietary Fiber

2.8g Sugars 7.7g Protein

142.   Egg drop soup

Preparation Time: 5 minutes

Cooking Time: 15 minutes

Servings: 2

Ingredients:

2 eggs, large

A pinch of red pepper flakes

4 cups bone broth

2 tablespoons scallions, sliced

Freshly ground pepper and salt to taste

Directions:

Scramble the eggs with some fresh pepper in a large bowl

set aside.

Now, over high heat settings in a small pot

add bone broth and a pinch of red pepper flakes. Bring it to a boil and then, slowly stir in the egg mixture

continue to mix and bring it to a boil again.

Remove from the stove

add pepper and salt to taste

Evenly divide the sliced scallions in half

garnish each bowl with it. Enjoy.

Nutrition:

78 Calories

6.1g Total Fat

3.3g Saturated Fat

3.5g Total Carbohydrates

0.7g Dietary Fiber

2.2g Sugars

6.1g Protein

143. French onion soup

Preparation Time: 10 minutes

Cooking Time: 50 minutes

Servings: 6

Ingredients:

4 drops of erythritol or stevia

1 ¼ oz. medium-sized brown onion

chopped

5 tablespoons butter

3 cups beef stock

4 tablespoons olive oil

Directions:

Over medium low heat in a pot

heat the olive oil and butter. Once the butter is melted

add the onions.

Cook until the onions turn golden brown, for 20 minutes, uncovered, stirring frequently. Stir in the stevia and cook for 5 more minutes.

Add stock to the saucepan

decrease the heat settings to low and let simmer for 25 more minutes.

Ladle the soup into separate soup bowls

serve immediately and enjoy.

Nutrition:

219 Calories

19g Total Fat

7.4g Saturated Fat

6g Total Carbohydrates

1.6g Dietary Fiber

4.7g Sugars

3.5g Protein

144. Cauliflower Faux-tatoes

Preparation Time: 10 minutes

Cooking Time: 5 minutes

Servings: 1

Ingredients:

3 oz. cauliflower

cored and cut into large chunks

¼ teaspoon garlic powder

1/2 tablespoon butter, optional

A handful of chives, optional

1 cup water

1/8 teaspoon each of pepper and salt

Directions:

Add steamer basket/trivet, water and cauliflower to the instant pot.

Cover your instant pot with a lid

set the valve to sealing.

Select the Manual setting and cook on high pressure for 3 to 5 minutes, less for a firmer mash.

Once done

immediately perform a quick release and carefully remove the lid.

Carefully remove the inner pot to drain water from and place the cauliflower to an empty and cleaned inner pot.

Add butter and the seasonings.

Puree the soup using an immersion blender until you get your desired consistency.

Give the ingredients a good stir

serve immediately and enjoy.

Nutrition:

87 Calories

7.6g Total Fat

3.9g Saturated Fat

3.1g Total Carbohydrates

2.1g Dietary Fiber

0.8g Sugars

1.5g Protein

145. Avocado soup

Preparation time: 15 minutes

Cooking time: 8 minutes

Servings: 4

Ingredients

4 cups homemade chicken broth

2 avocados

peeled, pitted, and chopped

1/3 cups fresh cilantro, chopped roughly

½ teaspoon garlic, chopped roughly

1 teaspoon fresh lime juice

Ground black pepper, to taste

½ pound cooked bacon, chopped

Directions:

In a large pan, add the broth over medium-high heat and bring to a boil.

Adjust the heat to low.

In a blender, add the avocadoes, cilantro, garlic, and lime juice, and pulse until chopped finely.

Add 1 cup of the chicken broth and pulse until smooth.

Transfer the avocado mixture into the pan of remaining simmering broth and stir to combine.

Stir in the salt and pepper and cook for about 2–3 minutes.

Top with bacon pieces and serve immediately.

Nutrition:

Calories 520

Net Carbs 3.2 g

Total Fat 41.7 g

Saturated Fat 11.7 g

Cholesterol 62 mg

Sodium 2,000 mg

Total Carbs 9 g

Fiber 5.8 g

Sugar 1.1 g

Protein 27.5 g

146. Egg drop soup

Preparation time: 10 minutes

Cooking time: 20 minutes

Servings: 6

Ingredients

1 tablespoon olive oil

1 tablespoon garlic, minced

6 cups homemade chicken broth, divided

2 organic eggs

1 tablespoon arrowroot powder

1/3 cup fresh lemon juice

Freshly ground white pepper, to taste

¼ cup scallion (green part), chopped

Directions:

In a large soup pan, heat the oil over medium-high heat and sauté garlic for about 1 minute.

Add 5½ cups of broth and bring to a boil over high heat.

Adjust the heat to medium and simmer for about 5 minutes.

Meanwhile, in a bowl, add eggs, arrowroot powder, lemon juice, white pepper, and remaining broth, and beat until well combined.

Slowly, add egg mixture in the pan, stirring continuously.

Simmer for about 5–6 minutes or until desired thickness of soup, stirring continuously

Serve hot with the garnishing of scallion.

Nutrition:

Calories 92

Net Carbs 3.2 g

Total Fat 5.3 g

Saturated Fat 1.3 g

Cholesterol 55 mg

Sodium 787 mg

Total Carbs 3.4 g

Fiber 0.2 g

Sugar 1.2 g

Protein 7 g

147. Tofu & spinach soup

Preparation time: 15 minutes

Cooking time: 35 minutes

Servings: 4

Ingredients

1 tablespoon olive oil

¼ cup onions, sliced thinly

3 garlic cloves, sliced

4 cups vegetable broth

1 tablespoon Sriracha

1 (4-inch piece) lemongrass, sliced and smashed

1 (5-ounces) package baby spinach

1 cup firm tofu

pressed, drained, and cut into ½-inch cubes

1 tablespoon fresh cilantro, chopped

3 tablespoons fresh lime juice

Directions:

In a heavy large pan, heat the oil over medium-low heat and cook the onions, garlic, and a little salt for about 15 minutes, stirring occasionally.

Stir in the broth, Leaping Sriracha, and lemongrass, and cover the pan.

Increase the heat to high and bring to a boil.

Remove from the heat and set aside, covered for about 15 minutes.

Uncover the pan and discard lemongrass.

In the pan, add the spinach, tofu, cilantro, and lime juice, and stir to combine.

Place the pan over medium heat and cook for about 3–4 minutes or until spinach is wilted, stirring occasionally.

Stir in the salt and remove from the heat.

Serve hot.

Nutrition:

Calories 132

Net Carbs 3.9 g

Total Fat 7.7 g

Saturated Fat 1.4 g

Cholesterol 0 mg

Sodium 826 mg

Total Carbs 5.5 g

Fiber 1.6 g

Sugar 1.6 g

Protein 11.3 g

148. Beef & mushroom soup

Preparation time: 15 minutes

Cooking time: 1 hour 20 minutes

Total time: 1 hour 35 minutes

Servings: 6

Ingredients

¼ cup olive oil

2 pounds grass-fed beef stew meat, cut into ½-inch chunks

½ cup yellow onion, chopped

2 garlic cloves, minced

1 teaspoon dried thyme, crushed

12 ounces fresh white mushrooms, sliced

2 cups fresh tomatoes, chopped finely

6 cups homemade chicken broth

3 tablespoons fresh lemon juice

¼ cup fresh cilantro, chopped

Salt and ground black pepper, to taste

Directions:

In a large pan, heat 2 tablespoons of oil over medium heat and sear the beef cubes in 2 batches for about 3–4 minutes or until browned completely.

With a slotted spoon, transfer the beef cubes into a bowl.

In the same pan, heat the remaining oil over medium heat and sauté the onion and garlic for about 2–3 minutes.

Add the mushrooms and cook for about 5–6 minutes, stirring occasionally.

Stir in the cooked beef cubes and remaining ingredients except for sour cream and bring to a boil.

Adjust the heat to low and cook for about 1 hour.

Stir in the lemon juice, cilantro, salt, and black pepper, and remove from the heat.

Serve hot.

Nutrition:

Calories 422

Net Carbs 5 g

Total Fat 19.6 g

Saturated Fat 5.2 g

Cholesterol 135 mg

Sodium 899 mg

Total Carbs 6.6 g

Fiber 1.6 g

Sugar 3.8 g

Protein 53.3 g

149.   Creamy chicken soup

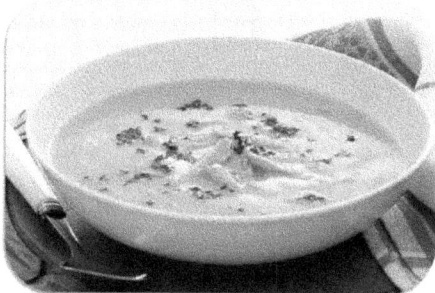

Preparation time: 15 minutes

Cooking time: 45 minutes

Total time: 1 hour

Servings: 4

Ingredients

1 tablespoon butter

1¼ cups tomatoes, chopped finely

3 Serrano peppers, chopped

1 tablespoon taco seasoning

1 pound grass-fed skinless, boneless chicken breasts

3¼ cups homemade chicken broth

8 ounces, cream cheese, softened

½ cup heavy cream

Salt, to taste

2 tablespoons fresh parsley, chopped

Directions:

In a Dutch oven, melt the butter over medium heat and cook the tomatoes, Serrano, and taco seasoning for about 1–2 minutes.

Add the chicken and broth and bring to a boil.

Adjust the heat to medium-low and simmer, covered for about 25 minutes.

With a slotted spoon, transfer the chicken breasts onto a plate.

With 2 forks, shred the meat.

In the pan of the soup, add the cream cheese and cream and cook for about 2–3 minutes, stirring continuously.

Remove from the heat and with an immersion blender, blend the soup until smooth.

Return the pan over medium heat and stir in the shredded chicken and salt.

Cook for about 1–2 minutes.

Stir in parsley and remove from the heat.

Serve hot.

Nutrition:

Calories 347

Net Carbs 4.4 g

Total Fat 14.2 g

Saturated Fat 7.3 g

Cholesterol 141 mg

Sodium 917 mg

Total Carbs 5.3 g

Fiber 0.9 g

Sugar 2.6 g

Protein 47.3 g

150. Coconut soup

Preparation time: 15 minutes

Cooking time: 35 minutes

Servings: 6

Ingredients:

1½ cups of coconut milk

4 cups chicken stock

1 tsp fried lemongrass

3 lime leaves

4 Thai chilies, dried and chopped

1-inch fresh ginger, peeled and grated

1 cup fresh cilantro, chopped

Salt and ground black pepper to taste

1 tbsp fish sauce

1 tbsp coconut oil

2 tbsp mushrooms, chopped

4 oz shrimp, peeled and deveined

2 tbsp onion, chopped

1 tbsp fresh cilantro, chopped

Juice from 1 lime

Directions:

In a medium pot, combine coconut milk, chicken stock, lemongrass, and lime leaves.

Preheat pot on medium heat.

Add Thai chilies, ginger, cilantro, salt, and pepper, stir and bring to simmer—Cook for 20 minutes.

Strain soup and return liquid to the pot.

Heat soup over medium heat.

Add fish sauce, coconut oil, mushrooms, shrimp, and onion. Stir well—Cook for 10 minutes.

Add cilantro and lime juice, stir. Set aside for 10 minutes.

Serve.

Nutrition:

Calories: 448

Carbohydrates: 7.9g

fat 33.8g

Protein: 11.8g

151. Broccoli soup

Preparation time: 12 minutes

Cooking time: 35 minutes

Servings: 4

Ingredients:

2 cloves garlic

1 medium white onion

1 tbsp butter

2 cups of water

2 cups vegetable stock

1 cup heavy cream

Salt and ground black pepper to taste

½ tsp paprika

1½ cups broccoli, divided into florets

1 cup cheddar cheese

Directions:

Peel and mince garlic. Peel and chop the onion.

Preheat pot on medium heat, add butter and melt it.

Add garlic and onion and sauté for 5 minutes, stirring occasionally.

Pour in water, vegetable stock, heavy cream, and add pepper, salt, and paprika.

Stir and bring to boil.

Add broccoli and simmer for 25 minutes.

After that, transfer soup mixture to a food processor and blend well.

Grate cheddar cheese and add to a food processor, blend again.

Serve soup hot.

Nutrition:

Calories: 348

Carbohydrates: 6.8g

fat 33.8g

Protein: 10.9g

152. Simple tomato soup

Preparation time: 15 minutes

Cooking time: 10 minutes

Servings: 6

Ingredients:

4 cups canned tomato soup

2 tbsp apple cider vinegar

1 tsp dried oregano

4 tbsp butter

2 tsp turmeric

2 oz red hot sauce

Salt and ground black pepper to taste

4 tbsp olive oil

8 bacon strips, cooked and crumbled

4 oz fresh basil leaves, chopped

4 oz green onions, chopped

Directions:

Pour tomato soup in the pot and preheat on medium heat. Bring to boil.

Add vinegar, oregano, butter, turmeric, hot sauce, salt, black pepper, and olive oil. Stir well.

Simmer the soup for 5 minutes.

Serve soup topped with crumbled bacon, green onion, and basil.

Nutrition:

Calories: 397 Carbohydrates: 9.8g

fat 33.8 Protein: 11.7g

153.   Green soup

Preparation time: 12 minutes

Cooking time: 15 minutes

Servings: 6

Ingredients:

2 cloves garlic

1 white onion

1 cauliflower head

2 oz butter

1 bay leaf, crushed

1 cup spinach leaves

½ cup watercress

4 cups vegetable stock

Salt and ground black pepper to taste

1 cup of coconut milk

½ cup parsley, for serving

Directions:

Peel and mince garlic. Peel and dice onion.

Divide cauliflower into florets.

Preheat pot on medium-high heat, add butter and melt it.

Add onion and garlic, stir, and sauté for 4 minutes.

Add cauliflower and bay leaf, stir and cook for 5 minutes.

Add spinach and watercress, stir and cook for another 3 minutes.

Pour in vegetable stock—season with salt and black pepper. Stir and bring to boil.

Pour in coconut milk and stir well. Take off heat.

Use an immersion blender to blend well.

Top with parsley and serve hot.

Nutrition:

Calories: 227 Carbohydrates: 4.89g

fat 35.1 Protein: 6.97g

154.   Sausage and Peppers Soup

Preparation time: 15 minutes

Cooking time: 1 hour 15 minutes

Servings: 6

Ingredients:

1 tbsp avocado oil

2 lbs pork sausage meat

Salt and ground black pepper to taste

1 green bell pepper, seeded and chopped

5 oz canned jalapeños, chopped

5 oz canned tomatoes, chopped

1¼ cup spinach

4 cups beef stock

1 tsp Italian seasoning

1 tbsp cumin

1 tsp onion powder

1 tsp garlic powder

1 tbsp chili powder

Directions:

Preheat pot with avocado oil on medium heat.

Put sausage meat in pot and brown for 3 minutes on all sides.

Add salt, black pepper, and green bell pepper and continue to cook for 3 minutes.

Add jalapeños and tomatoes, stir well and cook for 2 minutes more.

Toss spinach and stir again close lid and cook for 7 minutes.

Pour in beef stock, Italian seasoning, cumin, onion powder, chili powder, garlic powder, salt, and black pepper, stir well. Close lid again. Cook for 30 minutes.

When time is up, uncover the pot and simmer for 15 minutes more.

Serve hot.

Nutrition:

Calories: 531

Carbohydrates: 3.99g

fat 44.5g

Protein: 25.8g

155. Avocado soup

Preparation time: 12 minutes

Cooking time: 15 minutes

Servings: 4

Ingredients:

2 tbsp butter

2 scallions, chopped

3 cups chicken stock

2 avocados, pitted, peeled, and chopped

Salt and ground black pepper to taste

⅔ cup heavy cream

Directions:

Preheat pot on medium heat, add butter and melt it.

Toss scallions, stir and sauté for 2 minutes.

Pour in 2 ½ cups stock and bring to simmer—Cook for 3 minutes.

Meanwhile, peel and chop avocados.

Place avocado, ½ cup of stock, cream, salt, and pepper in a blender and blend well.

Add avocado mixture to the pot and mix well—Cook for 2 minutes.

Sprinkle with more salt and pepper, stir.

Serve hot.

Nutrition:

Calories: 329 Carbohydrates: 5.9g

fat 22.9g Protein: 5.8g

156.   Avocado and Bacon Soup

Preparation time: 15 minutes

Cooking time: 15 minutes

Servings: 6

Ingredients:

1-quart chicken stock

2 avocados, pitted

⅓ cup fresh cilantro, chopped

1 tsp garlic powder

Salt and ground black pepper to taste

Juice of ½ lime

½ lb bacon, cooked and chopped

Directions:

Pour chicken stock in a pot and bring to boil over medium-high heat.

Meanwhile, peel and chop the avocados.

Place avocados, cilantro, garlic powder, salt, black pepper, and lime juice in blender or food processor and blend well.

Add the avocado mixture in boiling stock and stir well.

Add bacon and season with salt and pepper to taste.

Stir and simmer for 3-4 minutes on medium heat.

Serve hot.

Nutrition:

Calories: 298 Carbohydrates: 5.98g

fat 22.8g Protein: 16.8g

157.   Roasted bell peppers soup

Preparation time: 15 minutes

Cooking time: 20 minutes

Servings: 6

Ingredients:

1 medium white onion

2 cloves garlic

2 celery stalks

12 oz roasted bell peppers, seeded

2 tbsp olive oil

Salt and ground black pepper to taste

1-quart chicken stock

2/3 cup water

¼ cup Parmesan cheese, grated

⅔ cup heavy cream

Directions:

Peel and chop onion and garlic. Chop celery and bell pepper. Preheat pot with oil on medium heat. Put garlic, onion, celery, salt, and pepper in the pot, stir and sauté for 8 minutes. Pour in chicken stock and water. Add bell peppers and stir. Bring to boil, close lid, and simmer for 5 minutes. Reduce heat if needed. When time is up, blend soup using an immersion blender. Add cream and season with salt and pepper to taste. Take off heat.

Serve hot with grated cheese.

Nutrition:

Calories: 180 Carbohydrates: 3.9g

fat 12.9g Protein: 5.9g

158. Spicy bacon soup

Preparation time: 15 minutes

Cooking time: 30 minutes

Servings: 6

Ingredients:

10 oz bacon, chopped

Salt to taste

1 tbsp olive oil

2/3 cup cauliflower, divided into florets

4 oz green bell pepper, seeded and chopped

1 jalapeno pepper, seeded and chopped

4 cups chicken stock

2 tbsp full-fat cream

1 tsp ground black pepper

1 tsp chili pepper

Directions:

In a bowl, combine bacon with salt.

Heat a pan over medium heat and cook bacon for 5 minutes, stirring constantly.

Remove bacon from pan and set aside.

Pour olive oil in a pan and add cauliflower, bell pepper, and jalapeno.

Cook veggies on high heat for 1 minute, stirring occasionally.

In a saucepan, mix bacon with vegetables. Pour in chicken stock. Stir.

Close lid and cook for 20-25 minutes.

Open the lid and add cream, stir.

Season with salt, black pepper, and chili pepper. Stir and cook for 5 minutes more.

Serve.

Nutrition:

Calories: 301

Carbohydrates: 3.9g

fat 23g

Protein: 19g

159. Italian sausage soup

Preparation time: 15 minutes

Cooking time: 35 minutes

Servings: 10

Ingredients:

1 tsp avocado oil

2 cloves garlic

1 medium white onion

1½ lbs hot pork sausage, chopped

8 cups chicken stock

1 lb radishes, chopped

10 oz spinach

1 cup heavy cream

6 bacon slices, chopped

Salt and ground black pepper to taste

A pinch of red pepper flakes

Directions:

Preheat pot on medium-high heat and add oil.

Peel and chop garlic and onion.

Put garlic, onion, and sausage in the pot and stir.

Cook for few minutes until browned.

Pour in chicken stock

add radishes and spinach, stir.

Bring mixture to simmer and add cream, bacon, black pepper, salt, and red pepper flakes, stir well.

Simmer for 20 minutes.

Serve hot.

Nutrition:

Calories: 289

Carbohydrates: 3.8g

fat 21.8g

Protein: 18.1g

CHAPTER 13:

Smoothies And Fresh Juices Recipes

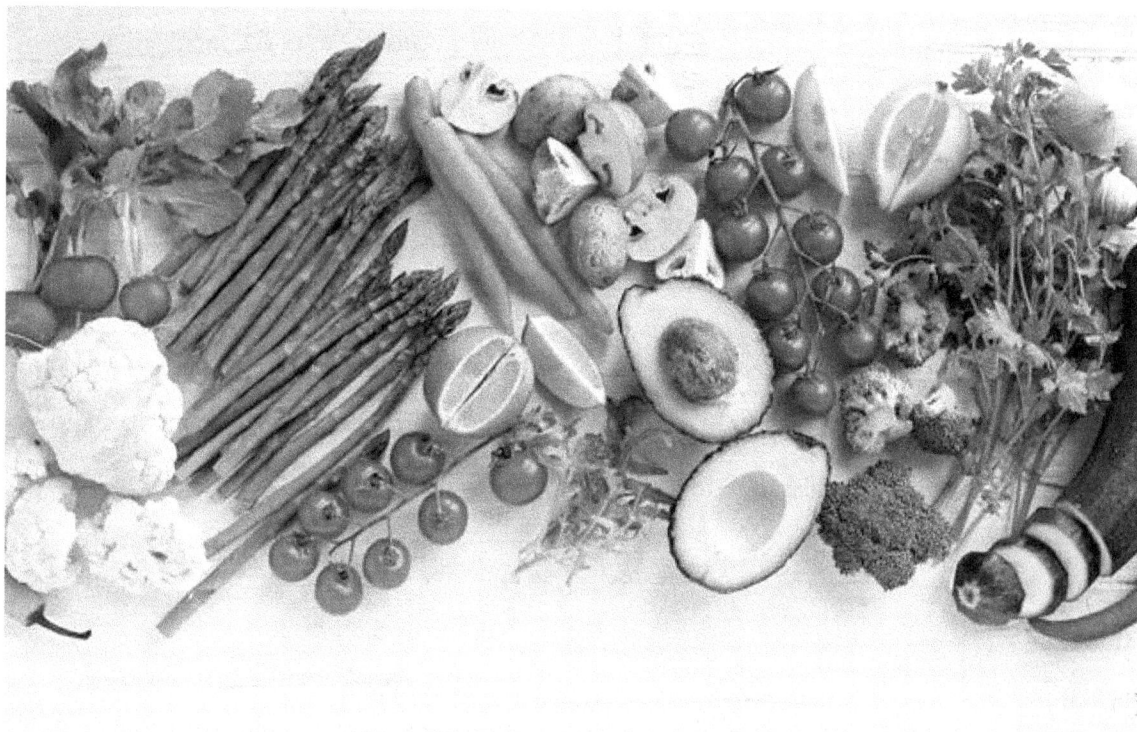

160. Almond smoothie

Preparation time: 10 minutes

Servings: 2

Ingredients

¾ cup almonds, chopped

½ cup heavy whipping cream

2 teaspoons butter, melted

¼ teaspoon organic vanilla extract

7–8 drops liquid stevia

1 cup unsweetened almond milk

¼ cup ice cubes

Directions:

In a blender, put all the listed ingredients and pulse until creamy.

Pour the smoothie into two glasses and serve immediately.

Nutrition:

Calories 365

Net Carbs 4.5 g

Total Fat 34.55 g

Saturated Fat 10.8 g

Cholesterol 51 mg

Sodium 129 mg

Total Carbs 9.5 g

Fiber 5 g

Sugar 1.6 g

Protein 8.7 g

161. Mocha smoothie

Preparation time: 10 minutes

Servings: 2

Ingredients

2 teaspoons instant espresso powder

2–3 tablespoons granulated erythritol

2 teaspoons cacao powder

½ cup plain Greek yogurt

1 cup unsweetened almond milk

1 cup ice cubes

Directions:

In a blender, put all the listed ingredients and pulse until creamy.

Pour the smoothie into two glasses and serve immediately.

Nutrition:

Calories 70

Net Carbs 5.5 g

Total Fat 2.8 g

Saturated Fat 1 g

Cholesterol 4 mg

Sodium 133 mg

Total Carbs 6.5 g

Fiber 1 g

Sugar 4.3 g

Protein 4.4 g

162. Strawberry smoothie

Preparation time: 10 minutes

Servings: 2

Ingredients

4 ounces frozen strawberries

2 teaspoons granulated erythritol

½ teaspoon organic vanilla extract

1/3 cup heavy whipping cream

1¼ cups unsweetened almond milk

½ cup ice cubes

Directions:

In a blender, put all the listed ingredients and pulse until creamy.

Pour the smoothie into two glasses and serve immediately.

Nutrition:

Calories 115

Net Carbs 4.5 g

Total Fat 9.8 g

Saturated Fat 4.8 g

Cholesterol 27 mg

Sodium 121 mg

Total Carbs 6.3 g

Fiber 1.8 g

Sugar 2.9 g

Protein 1.4 g

163. Raspberry smoothie

Preparation time: 10 minutes

Servings: 2

Ingredients

¾ cup fresh raspberries

3 tablespoons heavy whipping cream

1/3 ounce cream cheese

1 cup unsweetened almond milk

½ cup ice, crushed

Directions:

In a blender, put all the listed ingredients and pulse until creamy.

Pour the smoothie into two glasses and serve immediately.

Nutrition:

Calories 138

Net Carbs 3.8 g

Total Fat 12 g

Saturated Fat 6.4 g

Cholesterol 36 mg

Sodium 115 mg

Total Carbs 7.3 g

Fiber 3.5 g

Sugar 2.1 g

Protein 1.9 g

164. Pumpkin smoothie

Preparation time: 10 minutes

Servings: 2 Ingredients

½ cup homemade pumpkin puree

4 ounces cream cheese, softened

¼ cup heavy cream

½ teaspoon pumpkin pie spice

¼ teaspoon ground cinnamon

8 drops liquid stevia

1 teaspoon organic vanilla extract

1 cup unsweetened almond milk

¼ cup ice cubes

Directions:

In a blender, put all the listed ingredients and pulse until creamy.

Pour the smoothie into two glasses and serve immediately.

Nutrition:

Calories 296

Net Carbs 5.4 g

Total Fat 27.1 g

Saturated Fat 16.1g

Cholesterol 83 mg

Sodium 266 mg

Total Carbs 8 g

Fiber 2.6 g

Sugar 2.4 g

Protein 5.6 g

165. Spinach & avocado smoothie

Preparation time: 10 minutes

Servings: 2

Ingredients

½ large avocado, peeled, pitted, and roughly chopped

2 cups fresh spinach

1 tablespoon MCT oil

1 teaspoon organic vanilla extract

6–8 drops liquid stevia

1½ cups unsweetened almond milk

½ cup ice cubes

Directions:

In a blender, put all the listed ingredients and pulse until creamy.

Pour the smoothie into two glasses and serve immediately.

Nutrition:

Calories 180

Net Carbs 0 g

Total Fat 18 g

Saturated Fat 9 g

Cholesterol 0 mg

Sodium 161 mg

Total Carbs 6.5 g

Fiber 4.3 g

Sugar 0.6 g

Protein 2.4 g

166. Matcha smoothie

Preparation time: 10 minutes

Servings: 2

Ingredients

2 tablespoons chia seeds

2 teaspoons matcha green tea powder

½ teaspoon fresh lemon juice

½ teaspoon xanthan gum

10 drops liquid stevia

4 tablespoons plain Greek yogurt

1½ cups unsweetened almond milk

¼ cup ice cubes

Directions:

In a blender, put all the listed ingredients and pulse until creamy.

Pour the smoothie into two glasses and serve immediately.

Nutrition:

Calories 85

Net Carbs 3.5 g

Total Fat 5.5 g

Saturated Fat 0.8 g

Cholesterol 2 mg

Sodium 174 mg

Total Carbs 7.6 g

Fiber 4.1 g

Sugar 2.2 g

Protein 4 g

167. Creamy spinach smoothie

Preparation time: 10 minutes

Servings: 2

Ingredients

2 cups fresh baby spinach

1 tablespoon almond butter

1 tablespoon chia seeds

1/8 teaspoon ground cinnamon

Pinch of ground cloves

½ cup heavy cream

1 cup unsweetened almond milk

½ cup ice cubes

Directions:

In a blender, put all the listed ingredients and pulse until creamy.

Pour the smoothie into two glasses and serve immediately.

Nutrition:

Calories 195

Net Carbs 2.8 g

Total Fat 18.8 g

Saturated Fat 7.5 g

Cholesterol 41 mg

Sodium 126 mg

Total Carbs 6.1 g

Fiber 3.3 g

Sugar 0.5 g

Protein 4.5 g

168. Peanut butter cup smoothie

Preparation Time: 5 minutes

Cooking Time: 0 Minutes

Servings: 2

Ingredients:

1 cup water

¾ cup coconut cream

1 scoop chocolate protein powder

2 tablespoons natural peanut butter

3 ice cubes

Directions:

Put the water, coconut cream, protein powder, peanut butter, and ice in a blender and blend until smooth.

Pour into 2 glasses and serve immediately.

Nutrition:

Calories: 486

fat 40g

Protein: 30g

Carbs: 11g

Fiber: 5g

Net Carbs: 6g

Fat 70%

Protein 20%

Carbs 10%

169. Berry green smoothie

Preparation Time: 10 minutes

Cooking Time: 0 Minutes

Servings: 2

Ingredients:

1 cup water

½ cup raspberries

½ cup shredded kale

¾ cup cream cheese

1 tablespoon coconut oil

1 scoop vanilla protein powder

Directions:

Put the water, raspberries, kale, cream cheese, coconut oil, and protein powder in a blender and blend until smooth.

Pour into 2 glasses and serve immediately.

Nutrition:

Calories: 436

fat 36g

Protein: 28g

Carbs: 11g

Fiber: 5g

Net Carbs: 6g

Fat 70%

Protein 20%

Carbs 10%

170. Lemon-cashew smoothie

Preparation Time: 5 minutes

Cooking Time: 0 Minutes

Servings: 1

Ingredients:

1 cup unsweetened cashew milk

¼ cup heavy (whipping) cream

¼ cup freshly squeezed lemon juice

1 scoop plain protein powder

1 tablespoon coconut oil

1 teaspoon sweetener

Directions:

Put the cashew milk, heavy cream, lemon juice, protein powder, coconut oil, and sweetener in a blender and blend until smooth.

Pour into a glass and serve immediately.

Nutrition:

Calories: 503

fat 45g

Protein: 29g

Carbs: 15g

Fiber: 4g

Net Carbs: 11g

Fat 80%

Protein 13%

Carbs 7%

171. Spinach-blueberry smoothie

Preparation Time: 5 minutes

Cooking Time: 0 Minutes

Servings: 2

Ingredients: 1 cup spinach

1 cup coconut milk

½ English cucumber, chopped

½ cup blueberries

1 scoop plain protein powder

2 tablespoons coconut oil

4 ice cubes

Mint sprigs, for garnish

Directions:

Put the coconut milk, spinach, cucumber, blueberries, protein powder, coconut oil, and ice in a blender and blend until smooth.

Pour into 2 glasses, garnish each with the mint, and serve immediately.

Nutrition:

Calories:353

fat32g

Protein:15g

Carbs:9g

Fiber:3g

NetCarbs:6g

Fat76%/

Protein16%/

Carbs 8%

172. Creamy cinnamon smoothie

Preparation Time: 5 minutes

Cooking Time: 0 Minutes

Servings: 2

Ingredients:

2 cups coconut milk

1 scoop vanilla protein powder

5 drops liquid stevia

1 teaspoon ground cinnamon

½ teaspoon alcohol-free vanilla extract

Directions:

Put the coconut milk, protein powder, stevia, cinnamon, and vanilla in a blender and blend until smooth.

Pour into 2 glasses and serve immediately.

Nutrition:

Calories: 492

fat 47g

Protein: 18g

Carbs: 8g

Fiber: 2g

Net Carbs: 6g

Fat 80%/Protein 14%/Carbs 6%

CHAPTER 14:

Condiment, Sauces And Dressing Recipes

173. Curry powder

Preparation time: 10 minutes

Cooking time: 10 minutes

Servings: 20

Ingredients:

¼ cup coriander seeds

2 tablespoons mustard seeds

2 tablespoons cumin seeds

2 tablespoons anise seeds

1 tablespoon whole allspice berries

1 tablespoon fenugreek seeds

5 tablespoons ground turmeric

Directions:

In a large nonstick frying pan, place all the spices except turmeric over medium heat and cook for about 9–10 minutes or until toasted completely, stirring continuously.

Remove the frying pan from heat and set aside to cool.

In a spice grinder, add the toasted spices and turmeric, and grind until a subtle powder forms.

Transfer into an airtight jar to preserve.

Nutrition:

Calories 18

Net Carbs 1.8 g

Total Fat 0.8 g

Saturated Fat 0.1 g

Cholesterol 0 mg

Sodium 3 mg

Total Carbs 2.7 g

Fiber 0.9 g Sugar 0.1 g

Protein 0.8 g

174. Poultry seasoning

Preparation time: 5 minutes

Cooking time: 5 minutes

Servings: 10

Ingredients:

2 teaspoons dried sage, crushed finely

1 teaspoon dried marjoram, crushed finely

¾ teaspoon dried rosemary, crushed finely

1½ teaspoons dried thyme, crushed finely

½ teaspoon ground nutmeg

½ teaspoon ground black pepper

Directions:

Add all the ingredients in a bowl and stir to combine.

Transfer into an airtight jar to preserve.

Nutrition:

Calories 2

Net Carbs 0.2 g

Total Fat 0.1g

Saturated Fat 0.1 g

Cholesterol 0 mg

Sodium 0 mg   Total Carbs 0.4 g

Fiber 0.2 g   Sugar 0 g

Protein 0.1 g

175.   Bbq sauce

Preparation time: 15 minutes

Cooking time: 20 minutes

Servings: 20

Ingredients:

2½ (6-ounces) cans sugar-free tomato paste

½ cup organic apple cider vinegar

1/3 cup powdered erythritol

2 tablespoons Worcestershire sauce

1 tablespoon liquid smoke

2 teaspoons smoked paprika

1 teaspoon garlic powder

½ teaspoon onion powder

Salt, as required

¼ teaspoon red chili powder

¼ teaspoon cayenne pepper

1½ cups water

Directions:

Add all the ingredients (except the water) in a pan and beat until well combined.

Add 1 cup of water and beat until combined.

Add the remaining water and beat until well combined.

Place the pan over medium-high heat and bring to a gentle boil.

Adjust the heat to medium-low and simmer, uncovered for about 20 minutes, stirring frequently.

Remove the pan of sauce from the heat and set aside to cool slightly before serving.

You can preserve this sauce in refrigerator by placing it into an airtight container.

Nutrition:

Calories 22   Net Carbs 3.7 g

Total Fat 0.1 g

Saturated Fat 0 g

Cholesterol 0 mg

Sodium 46 mg

Total Carbs 4.7 g

Fiber 1 g

Sugar 3 g

Protein 1 g

176. Ketchup

Preparation time: 10 minutes

Cooking time: 30 minutes

Servings: 12

Ingredients:

6 ounces sugar-free tomato paste

1 cup of water

¼ cup powdered erythritol

3 tablespoons balsamic vinegar

½ teaspoon garlic powder

½ teaspoon onion powder

¼ teaspoon paprika

1/8 teaspoon ground cloves

1/8 teaspoon mustard powder

Salt, as required

Directions:

Add all ingredients in a small pan and beat until smooth.

Now, place the pan over medium heat and bring to a gentle simmer, stirring continuously.

Adjust the heat to low and simmer, covered for about 30 minutes or until desired thickness, stirring occasionally.

Remove the pan from heat and with an immersion blender, blend until smooth.

Now, set aside to cool completely before serving.

You can preserve this ketchup in the refrigerator by placing it in an airtight container.

Nutrition:

Calories 13

Net Carbs 2.3 g

Total Fat 0.1 g

Saturated Fat 0 g

Cholesterol 0 mg

Sodium 26 mg

Total Carbs 2.9 g

Fiber 0.6 g

Sugar 1.8 g

Protein 0.7 g

177. Cranberry sauce

Preparation time: 10 minutes

Cooking time: 15 minutes

Servings: 6

Ingredients:

12 ounces fresh cranberries

1 cup powdered erythritol

¾ cup of water

1 teaspoon fresh lemon zest, grated

½ teaspoon organic vanilla extract

Directions:

Place the cranberries, water, erythritol, and lemon zest in a medium pan and mix well.

Place the pan over medium heat and bring to a boil.

Adjust the heat to low and simmer for about 12–15 minutes, stirring frequently.

Remove the pan from heat and mix in the vanilla extract.

Set aside at room temperature to cool completely.

Transfer the sauce into a bowl and refrigerate to chill before serving.

Nutrition:

Calories 32

Net Carbs 3.2 g

Total Fat 0 g

Saturated Fat 0 g

Cholesterol 0 mg

Sodium 1 mg

Total Carbs 5.3 g

Fiber 2.1 g

Sugar 2.1 g

Protein 0 g

178. Yogurt tzatziki

Preparation time: 10 minutes

Cooking time: 0 minutes

Servings: 12

Ingredients:

1 large English cucumber, peeled and grated

Salt, as required

2 cups plain Greek yogurt

1 tablespoon fresh lemon juice

4 garlic cloves, minced

1 tablespoon fresh mint leaves, chopped

2 tablespoons fresh dill, chopped

Pinch of cayenne pepper

Ground black pepper, as required

Directions:

Arrange a colander in the sink.

Place the cucumber into the colander and sprinkle with salt.

Let it drain for about 10–15 minutes.

With your hands, squeeze the cucumber well.

Place the cucumber and remaining ingredients in a large bowl and stir to combine.

Cover the bowl and place in the refrigerator to chill for at least 4–8 hours before serving.

Nutrition:

Calories 36

Net Carbs 4.2 g

Total Fat 0.6 g

Saturated Fat 0.4 g

Cholesterol 2 mg

Sodium 42 mg

Total Carbs 4.5 g

Fiber 0.3 g

Sugar 3.3 g

Protein 2.7 g

179. American Jack Daniel's Sauce (Keto version)

Preparation Time: 10 minutes

Cooking Time: 25 minutes

Servings: 8

Ingredients:

1 cup water

2 tsp garlic minced

1 1/2 cups of natural granulated sweetener such Stevia

2 Tbsp of hot sauce

2 Tbsp of Coconut Aminos (soy sauce substitute

1 cup of lemon juice

1/4 cup of Jack Daniels Whiskey

2 Tbsp unsalted butter

1/4 tsp cayenne pepper

Directions:

In a small saucepan, pour the water, garlic, stevia sweetener, hot sauce and Cococnut aminos. Cook and stir over moderate heat for about 15 -20 minutes until sweetener dissolve, and the sauce thickens. Remove from heat and add the lemon juice, whiskey, butter and cayenne pepper stir well until sauce is smooth and shine. Let it cool and keep refrigerated in a glass container up to 3 months.

Nutrition:

Calories: 61 Carbohydrates 5g

proteins 1g fat 4g Fiber: 0.2g

180. Fresh mushroom sauce

Preparation Time: 10 minutes

Cooking Time: 15 minutes

Servings: 6

Ingredients:

1/4 cup of garlic-infused olive oil

1 tsp of garlic minced

1 lbs. fresh white mushrooms, sliced

1 cup of cherry tomatoes, cut into halves

1/2 cup green onions (scallions finely chopped

1/2 tsp salt and ground black pepper to taste

Directions:

Heat the olive oil in a frying skillet.

Add minced garlic along with mushrooms, and cook, stirring frequently, until mushroom liquid starts to evaporate, about 5 - 6 minutes.

Add cherry tomatoes, green onions, and season with the salt and black pepper.

Bring to boil, reduce heat, cover and cook for about 5 minutes or until the sauce is done.

Remove from heat and serve hot or cold.

Keep refrigerated in a covered glass bowl.

Nutrition:

Calories: 105

Carbohydrates 4g

proteins 3g

fat 10g Fiber: 1.3g

181. Spicy citrus bbq sauce

Preparation Time: 10 minutes

Cooking Time: 15 minutes

Servings: 6

Ingredients:

2 Tbsp of olive oil

1 large onion finely chopped

1/2 tsp ground red pepper (cayenne

1 chili pepper, seeded and finely chopped

1 1/2 cups lime juice (freshly squeezed

2 Tbsp of stevia granulate sweetener (or to taste

1 Tbsp of fresh cilantro finely chopped

1/4 tsp salt or to taste

Directions:

Heat the olive oil in a saucepan, and cook the onion, ground red pepper, and chili pepper, stirring frequently, until onion is tender, about 5 minutes. At this point, add all remaining Ingredients.

Bring to boil and reduce heat to the low

cook for further 10 minutes, stirring occasionally.

Remove the sauce from heat and allow it to cool.

Serve immediately or keep refrigerated.

Nutrition:

Calories: 61 Carbohydrates 6g

proteins 1g

fat 5g Fiber: 0.7g

182. Italian Pesto Dip with Ground Almonds

Preparation Time: 10 minutes

Cooking Time: 0 Minutes

Servings: 4

Ingredients:

2 cup of fresh basil

2 cloves of garlic minced

3 Tbsp of ground almonds, salted

3/4 cup extra virgin olive oil

1 Tbsp of lemon juice

Salt and ground black pepper

4 Tbsp of ground Parmesan cheese

Directions:

Place all Ingredients (except Parmesan in a food processor and pulse until well combined.

Add the parmesan cheese and pulse for 30 - 45 seconds.

Taste and adjust salt and pepper to taste.

Keep refrigerated.

Nutrition:

Calories: 426

Carbohydrates 3g

proteins 4g

fat 45g

Fiber: 1g

183. Keto "chimichurri" sauce

Preparation Time: 10 minutes

Cooking Time: 0 Minutes

Servings: 6

Ingredients:

1/2 cup of fresh oregano leaves, finely chopped

1/2 cup of fresh parsley, finely chopped

1/2 cup fresh cilantro, finely chopped

3 fresh bay leaves

2 jalapenos peppers, chopped

3 cloves garlic

1 Tbsp salt

1 Tbsp of chili powder

1/2 cup apple cider vinegar

1/2 cup of olive oil

Directions:

Add Ingredients from the list above in your food processor or blender.

Blend or process until smooth and all Ingredients are united well.

Serve immediately or keep refrigerated.

Nutrition:

Calories: 201

Carbohydrates 8g

proteins 1.2g

fat 19g Fiber: 4g

CHAPTER 15:

Appetizers & Beverages

184.   Iced keto coffee

Preparation Time: 5 Minutes

Cooking Time: -

Servings: 1

Ingredients

8 oz. cooled strongly brewed coffee.

1 scoop collagen peptides.

1 tablespoon Brain Octane Oil.

2 tablespoons original Nut pods.

Directions:

Add in ingredients like the coffee, collagen peptides and Brain Octane Oil to a medium glass then blend the ingredients together with the aid of a milk frother.

Add ice to the mixture then add the nut pods for taste. Stir and enjoy.

Nutrition:

Calories 191

Fats 16 g

Carbs 0.1 g

Proteins 10.1 g

185.   Jicama fries

Preparation Time: 45 minutes

Cooking time: 15 minutes

Servings: 2

Ingredients

1 jicama, peeled and sliced into thin strips

1/2 teaspoon onion powder

2 tablespoons avocado oil

Cayenne pepper, pinch

1 teaspoon paprika

Sea salt, to taste

Directions:

Dry roast the jicama strips in a non-stick frying pan (or you can also grease the pan with a bit of avocado oil). Place the roasted jicama fries into a large bowl and add the onion powder, cayenne pepper, paprika and sea salt. Drizzle over the avocado oil and toss the contents until the flavors are incorporated well. Serve immediately and enjoy!

Nutrition Info per Serving:

Calories 92 Fats 7 g

Proteins 1 g Carbs 2 g

186. Keto mocha

Preparation Time: 2 minutes

Cooking time: 5 minutes

Servings: 1

Ingredients:

2 shots espresso coffee

2 teaspoons of MCT oil

1 tablespoon of cocoa powder

2 teaspoons erythritol

2 tablespoons thick cream

1/2 cup of keto whipped cream

Directions:

Put the ingredients, MCT oil, cocoa powder and erythritol in a blender.

After blending, add a cup of boiling water.

Add cream and mix.

Serve hot and have fun!

Nutrition:

Calories 269 Fats 29 g

Carbs 1 g Proteins 1g

187. Keto turkish coffee

Preparation Time: 5 minutes

Cooking time: -

Servings: 1

Ingredients:

1 ½ tablespoons ground coffee beans

1 cup hot water

1 teaspoon of cardamom

½ cup of coconut milk

Stevia

Instruction:

Grind all the coffee beans and cardamom in a coffee grinder.

Pour the ground coffee and cardamom into the jar of a coffee maker.

Boil water.

Pour half of the water in the coffee jar.

Wait 30 seconds and mix the water and the ground coffee with a spoon.

Pour the rest of the hot water into the container and place the lid on the container.

Nutrition:

Calories 69

Fats 3 g

Carbs 0 g

Proteins 0g

188. Keto Ice Cream Coffee mix

Preparation Time: 10 minutes

Cooking Time: -

Servings: 1

Ingredients:

1 tablespoon of death wish coffee

1.5 cup vanilla milk without sugar

1 tablespoon of Keto MCT oil

1 tablespoon of chia seeds

2 tablespoons thick whipped cream

1 teaspoon vanilla extract.

2 teaspoon Stevia

Directions:

Freeze the coffee in an ice tray.

Put all ingredients in a blender and stir until smooth.

Pour in a glass. Before serving, wait 5 to 8 minutes for the chia seeds to thicken.

Nutrition:

Calories 344

Fats 32 g

Carbs 7 g

Proteins 4 g

189. Butter coffee

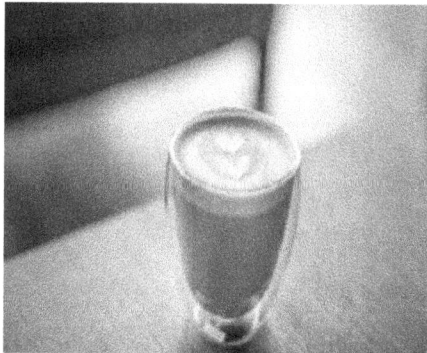

Preparation Time: 5 minutes

Cooking time: 5 minutes

Servings: 1

Ingredients

1 cup of water

2 tablespoons of coffee

1 tablespoon of herb-fed butter

1 tablespoon of coconut oil

Directions:

Make a cup of coffee your favorite way.

Simply simmer the ground coffee in the water for 5 minutes and filter it into a cup. You can also use a French press or a coffee machine!

Pour the brewed coffee, butter and coconut oil into the blender.

blend for about 10 seconds. You will see that it is immediately light and creamy!

Pour the coffee into a cup and enjoy! Add all other ingredients like cinnamon or whipped cream!

Nutrition:

Calories 230

Fats 25 g

Carbs 0 g

Proteins 0 g

190. Thai iced tea

Preparation Time: 2 minutes

Cooking time: 5 minutes

Servings: 1

Ingredients:

1 Thai teabag

½ cup of boiling water

6-8 ice cubes

¼ cup thick cream

8 drops of liquid stevia

Directions:

Soak a tea bag in 1/2 cup of boiled water for about 4 to minutes.

Take out the tea bag and pour the soaked tea into a glass to serve with 6-8 ice cubes.

Pour the thick cream and add liquid stevia. Mix everything and enjoy!

Nutrition:

Calories 205

Fats 21g

Carbs 1g

Proteins 1g

191.   Vanilla custard

Preparation Time: 10 minutes

Cooking time: 10 minutes

Servings: 2

Ingredients

8 egg yolks

1 cup unsweetened almond milk

1 teaspoon vanilla extract

10 stevia extract drops (optional)

6 tablespoons melted coconut oil or unsalted butter

Directions:

In a large, heatproof bowl, whisk the eggs, and then add the milk, vanilla, and honey.

Slowly mix in the melted coconut oil.

Now place this bowl over a pan of simmering water.

Insert a cooking thermometer into the pudding. Once the thermometer reads 140°F, remove the custard from the water bath.

Serve it warm or chilled.

Nutrition:

Calories 547

Fats 54 g

Carbs 4 g

Proteins 12 g

192.   Vanilla pana cotta

Preparation Time: 15 minutes

Cooking time: 5 minutes

Servings: 2

Ingredients:

1 teaspoon gelatin powder

1 tablespoon water

1 cup heavy whipping cream

½ tablespoon pure vanilla extract

1 tablespoon fresh pomegranate seeds

Directions:

Mix the gelatin powder with the water, and set it aside for 5 minutes.

Combine the cream and vanilla extract in a saucepan.

Bring the mixture to the boil, then lower the heat and let it simmer.

Once the cream begins to thicken, add the gelatin.

Stir until the gelatin is dissolved, and pour the cream into serving glasses.

Place it in the fridge for two hours, until it is completely cool.

Sprinkle the pomegranate seeds on top before serving.

Nutrition:

Calories 422

Fats 43 g

Carbs 4 g

Proteins 4 g

193. Creamy cinnamon coffee

Preparation Time: 10 minutes

Cooking time: 0 minutes

Servings: 2

Ingredients

4 tablespoons instant coffee

2 teaspoons ground cinnamon

2 cups boiling water

1 cup heavy whipping cream

Stevia liquid extract, optional

Directions:

Mix the coffee and cinnamon together.

Add the hot water, and stir.

Whip the cream until it is light and fluffy. Add a few drops of stevia if you like your coffee sweet.

Serve the coffee in a mug with the whipping cream on top.

Nutrition:

Calories 136 Fats 14 g

Carbs 2 g Protein 1 g

194. Chia seed pudding

Preparation Time: 5 minutes

Cooking time: 0 minutes

Servings: 2

Ingredients

1 ½ cup coconut milk

4 tablespoons Chia seeds

1 teaspoon pure vanilla extract

10 drops stevia extract

Directions:

Combine all the ingredients in a large jar.

Cover the jar and place it in the refrigerator to chill.

Once the pudding thickens and the chia seeds have gelled, serve the pudding with whipped cream.

Nutrition

Calories 186 Fats 13 g

Carbs 16 g Protein 7 g

195. Tasty chicken egg rolls
Preparation Time: 2 hours and 10 minutes

Cooking time: 15 minutes

Servings: 12

Ingredients:

4 ounces blue cheese

2 cups chicken, cooked and finely chopped

Salt and black pepper to the taste

2 green onions, chopped

2 celery stalks, finely chopped

½ cup tomato sauce

½ teaspoon erythritol

12 egg roll wrappers

Vegetable oil

Directions:

In a bowl, mix chicken meat with blue cheese, salt, pepper, green onions, celery, tomato sauce and sweetener, stir well and keep in the fridge for 2 hours.

Place egg wrappers on a working surface, divide chicken mix on them, roll and seal edges.

Heat up a pan with vegetable oil over medium high heat, add egg rolls, cook until they are golden, flip and cook on the other side as well.

Arrange on a platter and serve them.

Nutrition:

Calories 220 Fats 7 g

Carbs 6 g Protein 10 g

196. Avocado gazpacho
Preparation Time: 15 minutes

Servings: 2

Ingredients:

2 avocados, peeled, pitted and chopped

3 tablespoons fresh cilantro leaves

1½ cups homemade vegetable broth

1 tablespoon fresh lemon juice

½ teaspoon ground cumin

1/8 teaspoon cayenne pepper

Salt, as required

Directions:

Add all the ingredients in a high-speed blender and pulse until smooth.

Transfer the gazpacho into a large bowl.

Cover the bowl and refrigerate to chill completely before serving.

Nutrition:

Calories 235 Fats 20.7 g

Carbs 9.4 g Proteins 5.6 g

197. Spinach chips
Preparation Time: 5 minutes

Cooking time: 15 minutes

Servings: 6

Ingredients:

1 tablespoon olive oil

1-pound baby spinach

½ teaspoon curry powder

A pinch of salt and black pepper

½ teaspoon cumin, ground

Directions:

In a bowl, mix the spinach leaves with the oil and the other ingredients and toss gently.

Spread the basil leaves well on a baking sheet lined with parchment paper, and cook in the oven at 420 degrees F for 15 minutes.

Cool down and serve as a snack.

Nutrition:

Calories 30

Fats 3 g

Carbs 0.5 g

Protein 1 g

198. Parsley dip

Preparation Time: 5 minutes

Cooking time: 0 minutes

Servings: 6

Ingredients:

1 cup parsley

2 tablespoons pine nuts, toasted

2 tablespoons olive oil

3 ounces heavy cream

¼ teaspoon garlic powder

A pinch of salt and black pepper

1 chili pepper, chopped

Directions:

In a blender, combine the parsley with the pine nuts and the other ingredients, pulse well, divide into small bowls and serve as a dip.

Nutrition:

Calories 130

Fats 3.8 g

Carbs 2.2 g

Protein 5 g

CHAPTER 16:

Salad Recipes

199. Berries & spinach salad

Preparation time: 10 minutes

Servings: 5

Ingredients

Salad

8 cups fresh baby spinach

¾ cup fresh strawberries, hulled and sliced

¾ cup fresh blueberries

¼ cup onion, sliced

¼ cup almond, sliced

¼ cup feta cheese, crumbled

Dressing

1/3 cup olive oil

2 tablespoons fresh lemon juice

¼ teaspoon liquid stevia

1/8 teaspoon garlic powder

Salt, to taste

Directions:

For salad: In a bowl, add the spinach, berries, onion, and almonds, and mix.

For dressing: In another small bowl, add all the ingredients and beat until well combined.

Place the dressing over salad and gently, toss to coat well.

Nutrition:

Calories 190

Net Carbs 6 g

Total Fat 17.2 g

Saturated Fat 3.3 g

Cholesterol 7 mg

Sodium 145 mg

Total Carbs 8.5 g

Fiber 2.5 g

Sugar 4.6 g

Protein 3.3 g

200. Egg & avocado salad

Preparation time: 10 minutes

Servings: 4

Ingredients

Dressing

3 tablespoons olive oil

1 tablespoon fresh lime juice

Salt and ground black pepper, to taste

Salad

5 cups fresh baby greens

4 hard-boiled organic eggs, peeled and sliced

2 avocados

peeled, pitted, and sliced

2 tablespoons fresh mint leaves

Directions:

For dressing: Place oil, lime juice, salt, and black pepper in a small bowl and beat until well combined.

Divide the spinach onto serving plates and top each with tuna, egg, cucumber, and tomato.

Drizzle with dressing and serve.

Nutrition:

Calories 332 Net Carbs 2.5 g

Total Fat 31.5 g

Saturated Fat 6.4 g

Cholesterol 164 mg

Sodium 111 mg Total Carbs 8.8 g

Fiber 6.3 g Sugar 1.2 g

Protein 7.7 g

201. Tomato, arugula & mozzarella salad

Preparation time: 15 minutes

Servings: 4

Ingredients

Dressing

½ cup fresh basil leaves

2 garlic cloves, peeled

4 tablespoons olive oil

2 tablespoon balsamic vinegar

Salt and ground black pepper, to taste

Salad

2 cups cherry tomatoes

3 ounces mozzarella cheese balls

5 cups fresh arugula

Directions:

For dressing: In a small blender, add all the ingredients and pulse until smooth.

For salad: In a large bowl, add all the ingredients and mix.

Place the dressing over salad and toss to coat well.

Serve immediately.

Nutrition:

Calories 207

Net Carbs 4.2 g

Total Fat 18.1 g

Saturated Fat 4.3 g

Cholesterol 11 mg

Sodium 178 mg

Total Carbs 5.8 g

Fiber 1.6 g

Sugar 2.9 g

Protein 7.6 g

202. Smoked salmon & zucchini salad

Preparation time: 15 minutes

Servings: 6

Ingredients

Dressing

3 tablespoons olive oil

2 tablespoons balsamic vinegar

½ tablespoon Dijon mustard

¼ teaspoon red pepper flakes, crushed

Salad

12 ounces smoked salmon

3 medium zucchinis, spiralized with blade C

1 cup fresh mozzarella balls

2 tablespoons fresh basil, chopped

Directions:

For dressing: In a small blender, add all the ingredients and pulse until smooth.

For salad: In a large bowl, add all the ingredients and mix.

Place the dressing over salad and toss to coat well.

Serve immediately.

Nutrition:

Calories 158

Net Carbs 2.4 g

Total Fat 10.5 g

Saturated Fat 2.1 g

Cholesterol 16 mg

Sodium 1,100 mg

Total Carbs 3.6 g

Fiber 1.2 g

Sugar 1.7 g

Protein 13 g

203. Creamy shrimp salad

Preparation time: 15 minutes

Servings: 4

Ingredients

¼ cup sour cream

2 tablespoons mayonnaise

2 tablespoons fresh lemon juice

1 teaspoon Old Bay seasoning

Salt, to taste

16 ounces cooked shrimp

2 medium cucumbers, peeled and chopped

3 tablespoons fresh parsley, chopped

Directions:

Add sour cream, mayonnaise, lime juice, Old Bay, and salt in a large salad bowl and mix well.

Add remaining ingredients and gently, stir to combine.

Refrigerate to chill before serving.

Nutrition:

Calories 225

Net Carbs 4.9 g

Total Fat 10.1 g

Saturated Fat 3.3 g

Cholesterol 248 mg

Sodium 533 mg

Total Carbs 5.4 g

Fiber 0.5 g

Sugar 1.5 g

Protein 26.9 g

For a quick and easy meal, it is a great idea to have salads on hand. These can be staples in your diet, whether you are eating salad for lunch or dinner. If you incorporate any of these meals throughout the week, it can help you save time and stick to your diet on the busiest of days.

204. Pesto chicken salad

Preparation Time: 10 minutes

Cooking Time: Thirty Minutes

Servings: Four

Ingredients

Chicken Breast-4 Pieces]

Pesto-.50 CUPS

Cherry Tomatoes-1 CUPS

Spinach-3 CUPS

Salt-Dash]

Olive Oil-3 TBSP

Directions

For another alternative for plain old, baked chicken, you will want to consider this delicious Pesto chicken salad! To start off, you are going to want to go ahead and prep the stove to 350. As this warms up, place your chicken pieces onto a baking plate and coat with the pepper, salt, and olive oil. When this is done, pop the dish into the oven for forty minutes.

When the chicken is cooked through and no longer pink on the inside, you will now take it away from the oven and cool slightly before handling.

Once you can handle the chick, you will want to toss it into a bowl along with the pesto and your sliced tomatoes. When the ingredients are mended to your liking, place over a bowl of fresh spinach and enjoy your salad.

Nutrition

Fats: 12g

Carbs: 2g

Proteins: 40g

205. Fresh summer salad

Servings: Four

Preparation Time: 10 minutes

Cooking Time: 10 minutes

Ingredients

Olive Oil-2 TBSP

Thyme-1 tsp

Oregano-1 tsp

Ricotta Cheese-.25 CUPS

Basil-1 Leaf, Chopped]

Balsamic Vinegar-1 TBSP

Cucumber-1, Sliced]

Tomato-3, Sliced]

Radishes-5, Sliced]

Onion-1, Sliced]

Directions

Don't be fooled by the name

this salad can be enjoyed at any time of the year! If you are looking for a meatless dish, this is the perfect recipe for you! The first step you will want to take for this recipe will be making your ricotta cheese. You can complete this in a small bowl by mending the thyme, oregano, basil in with the ricotta cheese.

Next, you will be making your own dressing! For this task, all you have to do is whisk your vinegar and olive oil together. Once this is complete, season however you would like.

Finally, take some time to slice and dice the vegetables according to the directions above. When your veggies are all set, you will want to assemble them in your serving dishes and pour the dressing generously over the top. As a final touch, dollop your ricotta cheese over your salad, and then your salad will be ready for serving.

Nutrition

Fats: 10g

Carbs: 8g

Proteins: 5g

206. Keto taco salad

Preparation Time: 10 minutes

Cooking Time: Twenty Minutes

Servings: Six

Ingredients

Ground Beef-1 Ln.

Olive Oil-3 TBSP

Pepper-Dash]

Onion Powder-1 TBSP

Cumin-1 TBSP

Garlic Clove-1 T., Minced]

Tomato-1, Chopped]

Sour Cream-.50 CUPS

Black Olives-.50 CUPS

Cheddar Cheese-.25 CUPS

Cilantro-2 TBSP

Green Pepper-1, Chopped]

Directions

With taco salad, you will be able to enjoy everything that you love about tacos with a lot less carbohydrates! Whether you prepare this for taco Tuesday or a quick lunch, it is sure to be a crowd-pleaser!

Start this recipe off by taking out your grilling pan and place it over a moderate temperature. As it warms up, you can add in the olive oil and let that sizzle. When you are set, add in the green pepper, spices, and ground beef. You can also use ground turkey in this recipe if that is more your style. Go ahead and cook these ingredients together for 10 minutes or so.

When you are all set, place some mixed greens into a bowl and cover with the meat mixture you just created. If you would like some extra flavor, sprinkle some cheddar cheese over the top along with some sour cream.

Nutrition

Fats: 20g

Carbs: 5g

Proteins: 20g

207. Mixed vegetable tuna salad

Preparation Time: 10 minutes

Cooking Time: 10 minutes

Servings: Four

Ingredients

Canned Tuna-1 Can]

Olive Oil-2 TBSP

Parsley-.25 CUPS

Red Pepper-1, Roasted & Chopped]

Artichoke Hearts-.50 C., Diced]

Black Olives-.25 CUPS

Basil-2 TBSP

Lemon Juice-2 T.}

Pepper-Dash]

Directions

When you are in a rush, you can't go wrong with tuna salad! To save yourself even more time, you can go ahead and prep this tuna

salad at the beginning of the week so that all you will have to do is grab and go!

For this recipe, get out a mixing bowl and mend all of the items from the list above. Once combined, feel free to season with pepper and salt to your liking.

For serving purposes, this tuna salad can be enjoyed in a number of different ways. You can eat it right out of the bowl, scooped into a lettuce wrap, or served over a bed of salad!

Nutrition

Fats: 15g

Carbs: 3g

Proteins: 10g

208. Lemon shrimp salad

Preparation Time: 10 minutes

Cooking Time: Twenty Minutes

Servings: Four

Ingredients

Mixed Greens-5 CUPS

Olive Oil-2 TBSP

Shrimp-1 Lb.

Sliced Almonds-.25 CUPS

Avocado-2, Sliced]

Pepper-Dash]

Lemon Juice-2 TBSP

Directions

When people think about making a salad for lunch, they often think of either chicken or steak over the top. Have you ever considered shrimp on your salad? It is an awesome alternative when you don't feel like having chicken or steak again. To begin this recipe, you will first need to sear your shrimp.

For some added flavor, go ahead and mix your shrimp with some pepper and lemon juice. When it is coated to your liking, you are going to place it into a grilling pan over a moderate temperature. We are only going to sear the shrimp so it should only take two to three minutes on either side. You will just want to make sure that the shrimp is cooked thoroughly.

When the shrimp is cooked to your liking, it is time to assemble your salad. Go ahead and place your mixed greens into your serving bowls and squeeze some lemon juice over the top. Once these items are in place, add in the olive oil and begin layering the avocado on top.

For a final touch, add in the shrimp and sliced almonds for a bit of a crunch. Just like that, your salad will be fresh and ready for serving.

Nutrition

Fats: 30g

Carbs: 10g

Proteins: 30g

209. Potluck lamb salad

Preparation Time: 20 minutes

Cooking Time: 10 minutes

Servings: 4

Ingredients:

2 tbsp. olive oil, divided

12 oz. grass-fed lamb leg steaks, trimmed

Salt and freshly ground black pepper, to taste

6½ oz. halloumi cheese, cut into thick slices

2 jarred roasted red bell peppers, sliced thinly

2 cucumbers, cut into thin ribbons

3 C. fresh baby spinach

2 tbsp. balsamic vinegar

Directions:

In a skillet, heat 1 tbsp. of the oil over medium-high heat and cook the lamb steaks for about 4-5 minutes per side or until desired doneness.

Transfer the lamb steaks onto a cutting board for about 5 minutes.

Then cut the lamb steaks into thin slices.

In the same skillet, add haloumi and cook for about 1-2 minutes per side or until golden.

In a salad bowl, add the lamb, haloumi, bell pepper, cucumber, salad leaves, vinegar, and remaining oil and toss to combine.

Serve immediately.

Nutrition:

Calories: 420

Carbohydrates: 8g

Protein: 35.4g

fat 27.2g

Sugar: 4g

Sodium: 417mg

Fiber: 1.3g

210. Spring supper salad

Preparation Time: 15 minutes

Cooking Time: 5 minutes

Servings: 5

Ingredients:

For Salad:

1 lb. fresh asparagus, trimmed and cut into 1-inch pieces

½ lb. smoked salmon, cut into bite-sized pieces

2 heads red leaf lettuce, torn

¼ C. pecans, toasted and chopped

For Dressing:

¼ C. olive oil

2 tbsp. fresh lemon juice

1 tsp. Dijon mustard

Salt and freshly ground black pepper, to taste

Directions:

In a pan of boiling water, add the asparagus and cook for about 5 minutes. Drain the asparagus well. In a serving bowl, add the asparagus and remaining salad ingredients and mix. In another bowl, add all the dressing ingredients and beat until well combined. Place the dressing over salad and gently, toss to coat well. Serve immediately.

Nutrition:

Calories 223 Carbohydrates: 8.5g

Protein: 11.7g fat 17.2g Sugar: 3.4g

Sodium: 960mg Fiber: 3.5g

211. Chicken-of-Sea Salad

Preparation Time: 15 minutes

Cooking Time: 5 minutes

Servings: 6

Ingredients:

2 (6-oz.) cans olive oil-packed tuna, drained

2 (6-oz.) cans water packed tuna, drained

¾ C. mayonnaise

2 celery stalks, chopped

¼ of onion, chopped

1 tbsp. fresh lime juice

2 tbsp. mustard

Freshly ground black pepper, to taste

6 C. fresh baby arugula

Directions:

In a large bowl, add all the ingredients except arugula and gently stir to combine.

Divide arugula onto serving plates and top with tuna mixture.

Serve immediately.

Nutrition:

Calories: 325

Carbohydrates: 2.7g

Protein: 27.4g

fat 22.2g

Sugar: 0.9g

Sodium: 389mg

Fiber: 1.1g

212. Yummy roasted cauliflower

Preparation Time: 15 minutes

Cooking Time: 20 minutes

Servings: 5

Ingredients:

4 C. cauliflower florets

4 small garlic cloves, peeled and halved

2 tbsp. olive oil

1 tbsp. fresh lemon juice

1 tsp. dried thyme, crushed

1 tsp. dried oregano, crushed

½ tsp. red pepper flakes, crushed

Salt and freshly ground black pepper, to taste

Directions:

Preheat the oven to 425 degrees F. Generously, grease 2 large baking dishes.

In a large bowl, add all the ingredients and toss to coat well.

Divide the cauliflower mixture into the prepared baking dishes evenly and spread in a single layer.

Roast for about 15-20 minutes or until the desired doneness, tossing 2 times.

Remove from the oven and serve hot.

Nutrition:

Calories 74 Carbohydrates: 5.5g

Protein: 1.8g fat 5.8g

Sugar: 2g Sodium: 56mg

Fiber: 2.3g

213. Cheesy cauliflower mash

Preparation Time: 15 minutes

Cooking Time: 12 minutes

Servings: 6

Ingredients:

1 large head cauliflower, cut into florets

1/3 C. heavy whipping cream

1 C. Parmesan cheese, shredded and divided

1 tbsp. butter

Freshly ground black pepper, to taste

1 tbsp. fresh parsley, chopped

Directions:

In a large pan of boiling water, add the cauliflower and cook, covered for about 10-12 minutes.

Drain the cauliflower well.

In a large food processor, place the cauliflower, cream, ½ C. of cheese, butter, and black pepper and pulse until smooth.

Transfer the cauliflower mash into a bowl.

Top with the remaining cheese and parsley and serve.

Nutrition:

Calories: 107

Carbohydrates: 3g

Protein: 6.1g

fat 8.1g Sugar: 1.1g

Sodium: 256mg

Fiber: 1.1g

214. Buttered broccoli

Preparation Time: 10 minutes

Cooking Time: 15 minutes

Servings: 4

Ingredients:

2 medium heads broccoli, cut into florets

2 garlic cloves, minced

¼ C. butter, melted

2 tbsp. fresh lemon juice

1 tsp. Italian seasoning

Salt and freshly ground black pepper, to taste

Directions:

Preheat the oven to 450 degrees F.

In a bowl, add all ingredients and toss to coat well.

Place broccoli mixture into a large baking dish and spread in a single layer.

Bake for about 12-15 minutes.

Serve hot.

Nutrition:

Calories 109

Carbohydrates: 7.4g

Protein: 3.1g

fat 12.3g

Sugar: 2g

Sodium: 155mg

Fiber: 2.6g

215. Great side dish

Preparation Time: 10 minutes

Cooking Time: 15 minutes

Servings: 3

Ingredients:

2 C. broccoli florets

1 small yellow onion, cut into wedges

½ tsp. garlic powder

1/8 tsp. paprika

Freshly ground black pepper, to taste

2 tbsp. butter, melted

Directions:

Preheat the grill to medium heat.

In a large bowl, add all ingredients and toss to coat well.

Transfer the broccoli mixture over a double thickness of a foil paper.

Fold the foil around the broccoli mixture to seal it.

Grill for about 10-15 minutes.

Serve hot.

Nutrition:

Calories 99

Carbohydrates: 6.5g

Protein: 2.1g fat 7.9g

Sugar: 2.1g

Sodium: 76mg

Fiber: 2.1g

216. Appealing broccoli mash

Preparation Time: 15 minutes

Cooking Time: 5 minutes

Servings: 6

Ingredients:

16 oz. broccoli florets

1 C. water

1 tsp. fresh lemon juice

1 tsp. butter, softened

1 tsp. garlic, minced

Salt and freshly ground black pepper, to taste

Directions:

In a medium pan, add the broccoli and water over medium heat and cook for about 5 minutes.

Drain the broccoli well and transfer into a large bowl

In the bowl of broccoli, add the lemon juice, butter, and garlic and with an immersion blender blend until smooth.

Season with salt and black pepper and serve.

Nutrition:

Calories 32

Carbohydrates: 5.1g

Protein: 2g

fat 0.9g

Sugar: 1.3g

Sodium: 160mg

Fiber: 2g

217. Zesty brussels sprout

Preparation Time: 15 minutes

Cooking Time: 15 minutes

Servings: 2

Ingredients:

½ lb. fresh Brussels sprouts, trimmed and halved

2 tbsp. olive oil

2 small garlic cloves, minced

½ tsp. red pepper flakes, crushed

Salt and freshly ground black pepper, to taste

1 tbsp. fresh lemon juice

1 tsp. fresh lemon zest, grated finely

Directions:

Arrange a steamer basket over a large pan of the boiling water.

Place the asparagus into the steamer basket and steam, covered for about 6-8 minutes.

Remove from the heat and drain the asparagus well. In a large skillet, heat the oil over medium heat and sauté the garlic and red pepper flakes for about 1 minute. Stir in the Brussels sprouts, salt, and black pepper and sauté for about 4-5 minutes. Stir in the lemon juice and sauté for about 1 minute more. Remove from the heat and serve hot with the garnishing of the lemon zest.

Nutrition:

Calories: 116 Carbohydrates: 11g

Protein: 4.1g fat 7.5g Sugar: 2.5g

Sodium: 102mg Fiber: 4.4g

218.   Simplest yellow squash

Preparation Time: 10 minutes

Cooking Time: 12 minutes

Servings: 4

Ingredients:

2 tbsp. olive oil

1 lb. yellow squash, cut into thin slices

1 small yellow onion, cut into thin rings

1 garlic clove, minced

3 tsp. water

Salt and freshly ground white pepper, to taste

Directions:

In a large skillet, heat the oil over medium-high heat and stir fry the squash, onion, and garlic for about 3-4 minutes.

Add water, salt and black pepper and stir to combine.

Reduce heat to low and simmer for about 6-8 minutes.

Serve hot.

Nutrition:

Calories: 86

Carbohydrates: 5.7g

Protein: 1.6g

fat 7.2g

Sugar: 2.7g

Sodium: 51mg

Fiber: 1.7g

CHAPTER 17:

Snack Recipes

219. Tuscan truffles

Cooking Time: 25 minutes

Preparation Time: 10 minutes

Servings: 6

Ingredients

Two logs of goat cheese

Eight ounces of mascarpone cheese

Six tbsps. of parmesan cheese (grated)

Three cloves of garlic (minced)

Two tsps. of olive oil

One tsp. of white balsamic vinegar

Three-fourth tsp. of lemon zest (grated)

Six and a half tbsp. of prosciutto (chopped)

Five tbsps. of dried figs (chopped)

Three tbsps. of parsley (minced)

One-fourth tsp. of pepper

One cup of pine nuts (chopped)

Directions:

Mix the first eleven listed ingredients in a large bowl.

Shape the mixture into thirty-six small balls.

Roll the balls in chopped pine nuts.

Refrigerate for twenty minutes.

Nutrition: Calories: 82.3

Protein: 3.3g

Carbs: 1.6g

fat 7.3g

Fiber: 0.6g

220. Caprese salad kabobs

Cooking Time: 10 minutes

Preparation Time: 10 minutes

Servings: 4

Ingredients

Twenty-four grape tomatoes

Twelve small bits of mozzarella cheese balls

Twenty-four basil leaves.

Two tbsps. of olive oil

Two tsps. of balsamic vinegar

Directions:

Combine vinegar along with olive oil in a small bowl.

Thread two tomatoes, two leaves of basil, and one ball of cheese alternately on each skewer.

Drizzle the mixture of olive oil over the skewers.

Serve immediately.

Nutrition: Calories: 45.4

Protein: 2.3g

Carbs: 1.6g

fat 5.1g

Fiber: 1.2g

221. Roasted Cauliflower and Tahini Yogurt Sauce

Cooking Time: 45 minutes

Preparation Time: 10 minutes

Servings: 4

Ingredients

One-fourth cup of parmesan cheese (grated)

Three tbsps. of olive oil

Two cloves of garlic (minced)

One-fourth tsp. of salt

One-third tsp. of pepper

One cauliflower (cut in four wedges)

For the sauce:

Half cup of Greek yogurt

One tbsp. of lemon juice

Half tbsp. of tahini

One-fourth tsp. of salt

One pinch of paprika

Parsley (minced)

Directions:

Preheat your oven at one hundred and fifty degrees Celsius.

Mix the first five ingredients.

Rub the mixture over the wedges of cauliflower.

Grease a baking tray with cooking spray.

Arrange the wedges of cauliflower on the baking tray. Roast for forty minutes.

For the sauce, combine lemon juice, yogurt, seasonings, and tahini in a bowl.

Serve the cauliflower wedges and drizzle tahini sauce on top. Garnish with parsley.

Nutrition: Calories: 179.6

Protein: 7.6g

Carbs: 5.1g

fat 15.4g

Fiber: 2.2g

222. Zucchini crusted pizza

Cooking Time: 45 minutes

Preparation Time: 10 minutes

Servings: 6

fat 11.6g

Fiber: 1.6g

Ingredients

Two large eggs (beaten)

Two cups of zucchini (shredded, squeezed)

Half cup of mozzarella cheese (shredded)

One-third cup of parmesan cheese (grated)

One-fourth cup of flour

One tbsp. of olive oil

One and a half tbsp. of basil (minced)

One tsp. of thyme (minced)

For the toppings:

Twelve ounces of sweet red pepper (roasted, julienned)

One cup of mozzarella cheese (shredded)

Half cup of turkey pepperoni (sliced)

Directions:

Preheat your oven at two hundred degrees Celsius.

Combine the first eight listed ingredients in a bowl.

Transfer the mixture to a greased pizza pan. Spread the mixture and evenly press it to the base.

Bake for sixteen minutes.

Add the toppings on the pizza. Bake for twelve minutes.

Slice the pizza using a pizza cutter.

Serve hot.

Nutrition: Calories: 226.3

Protein: 13.6g

Carbs: 8.6g

223. Stuffed basil-asiago mushrooms

Cooking Time: 35 minutes

Preparation Time: 10 minutes

Servings: 4

Ingredients

Twenty-four Portobello mushrooms (remove the stems)

Half cup of mayonnaise

Three-fourth cup of Asiago cheese(shredded)

One-third cup of basil leaves (remove the stems)

One-fourth tsp. of white pepper

Twelve cherry tomatoes (halved)

Directions:

Preheat your oven at one hundred and fifty degrees Celsius.

Grease a baking dish with cooking spray.

Arrange the mushroom caps in the dish. Bake the mushrooms for 10 minutes .

Combine Asiago cheese, mayonnaise, pepper, and basil in a food processor. Mix well.

Fill the mushroom caps with the cheese and basil mixture. Top each mushroom cap with half a tomato.

Bake for 10 minutes .

Serve warm.

Nutrition:

Calories: 36.6 Protein: 2.3g Carbs: 1.5g

fat 3.3g Fiber: 0.3g

224. Cheese and Zucchini Roulades

Cooking Time: 25 minutes

Preparation Time: 10 minutes

Servings: 6

Ingredients

One cup of ricotta cheese

One-fourth cup of parmesan cheese (grated)

Two tbsps. of basil (minced)

One tbsp. of capers

One and a half tbsp. of Greek olives (chopped)

One tsp. of lemon zest (grated)

Two tbsps. of lemon juice

One-eighth tsp. of pepper

One-fourth tsp. of salt

Four zucchinis

Directions:

Combine the first nine listed ingredients in a bowl. Slice the zucchinis into twenty-four slices lengthwise. Grease a grill rack with cooking spray. Cook the slices of zucchini for three minutes.

Add one tbsp. of the ricotta cheese mixture on one end of the zucchini slices. Roll up the slices. Secure using toothpicks. Serve immediately.

Nutrition:

Calories: 29.4 Protein: 3.5g Carbs: 1.2g

fat 1.6g Fiber: 0.2g

225. Chicken nuggets with sweet potato crusting

Cooking Time: Thirty minutes

Preparation Time: 10 minutes

Servings: 4

Ingredients

One cup of sweet potato chips

One-fourth cup of flour

One tsp. of salt

Half tsp. of ground pepper (ground)

One-fourth tsp. of baking powder

One tbsp. of cornstarch

One pound of chicken tenderloins (cut in pieces of half-inch)

Oil (to fry)

Directions:

Heat the oil in a large skillet.

Add flour, chips, salt, baking powder, and pepper in a food processor. Pulse the ingredients for making a ground mixture.

Toss the chicken pieces in cornstarch. Shake off excess cornstarch. Toss in the chip mixture. Press the chicken pieces gently for coating.

Fry the chicken nuggets for three minutes.

Serve hot.

Nutrition:

Calories: 305.6 Protein: 26.6g Carbs: 8.6g

fat 18.9g Fiber: 1.6g

226. Artichoke and Spinach Stuffed Mushrooms

Cooking Time: Forty minutes

Preparation Time: 10 minutes

Servings: 6

Ingredients

Three ounces of cream cheese

Half cup of mayonnaise

One cup of sour cream

Three-fourth tsp. of garlic salt

One can of artichoke hearts (chopped)

Ten ounces of spinach (chopped)

One-third cup of mozzarella cheese (shredded)

Three tbsps. of parmesan cheese (shredded)

Thirty large mushrooms (remove the stems)

Directions:

Preheat your oven at two hundred degrees Celsius. Combine the first four listed ingredients in a bowl. Add spinach, artichoke, three tbsps. of parmesan cheese, and mozzarella cheese. Arrange the mushrooms on a large aluminum foil-lined baking tray. Add one tbsp. of the filling into the mushroom caps. Sprinkle remaining parmesan cheese from the top. Bake for twenty minutes.

Nutrition:

Calories: 52.2 Protein: 2.6g

Carbs: 1.5gfat 5.6g Fiber: 0.2g

227. Cobb salad sausage lettuce wraps

Cooking Time: 25 minutes

Preparation Time: 10 minutes

Servings: 6

Ingredients

Three-fourth cup of ranch salad dressing

One-third cup of blue cheese (crumbled)

One-fourth cup of watercress (chopped)

One pound of pork sausage

Two tbsps. of chives (minced)

Six leaves of iceberg lettuce

One avocado (peeled, diced)

Four boiled eggs (chopped)

One tomato (chopped)

Directions:

Combine blue cheese, dressing, and watercress in a bowl.

Heat some oil in an iron skillet. Add the sausage. Cook for seven minutes and crumble. Add the chives.

Spoon the sausage mixture into the leaves of lettuce. Top the sausage mixture with eggs, tomato, and avocado. Drizzle the mixture of dressing on top.

Serve immediately.

Nutrition:

Calories: 430.6 Protein: 16.5g Carbs: 5.8g

fat 39.6g Fiber: 3.5g

228. Mushroom and Asparagus Frittata

Cooking Time: 45 minutes

Preparation Time: 10 minutes

Servings: 8

Ingredients

Eight large eggs

Half cup of ricotta cheese

Two tbsps. of lemon juice

Half tsp. of salt

One-fourth tsp. of pepper

One tbsp. of olive oil

Eight ounces of asparagus spears

One onion (sliced)

One-third cup of sweet green pepper

Three-fourth cup of Portobello mushrooms (sliced)

Directions:

Preheat your oven at one hundred and fifty degrees Celsius.

Combine ricotta cheese, eggs, pepper, lemon juice, and salt in a bowl.

Heat oil in an iron skillet. Add onion, asparagus, mushrooms, and red pepper. Cook for eight minutes. Remove the asparagus from the skillet.

Cut the spears of asparagus into pieces of two-inch. Return the spears to the skillet.

Add the mixture of eggs.

Bake in the oven for twenty minutes.

Let the frittata sit for five minutes.

Cut the frittata into wedges. Serve warm.

Nutrition: Calories: 132.3

Protein: 9.3g

Carbs: 5.1g

fat 8.2g

Fiber: 1.6g

229. Sausage balls

Cooking Time: 45 minutes

Preparation Time: 10 minutes

Servings: 6

Ingredients

One pound of spicy pork sausage (ground)

Eight ounces of cream cheese

Half cup of cheddar cheese (shredded)

One-third cup of parmesan cheese (shredded)

One tbsp. of Dijon mustard

Half tsp. of garlic powder

One-fourth tsp. of salt

Directions:

Preheat your oven at one hundred and seventy degrees Celsius.

Use parchment paper for lining a baking sheet.

Combine cream cheese, sausage, parmesan cheese, cheddar cheese, garlic powder, mustard, and salt in a mixing bowl. Mix well.

Take one tbsp. of the mixture. Roll it into a ball. Repeat for the remaining mixture.

Arrange the prepared balls on the lined baking tray.

Bake for thirty minutes.

Serve hot.

Nutrition: Calories: 102.3

Protein: 5.9g

Carbs: 0.7g

fat 9.6g

Fiber: 0.2g

230. Ranch cauliflower crackers

Cooking Time: One hour and 10 minutes

Preparation Time: 10 minutes

Servings: 6

Ingredients

Twelve ounces of cauliflower rice

Cheesecloth

One large egg

One tbsp. of ranch salad dressing mix (dry)

One-eighth tsp. of cayenne pepper

One cup of parmesan cheese (shredded)

Directions:

Add the cauliflower rice in a large bowl. Microwave for four minutes covered.

Transfer the cauliflower rice to a strainer lined with cheesecloth. Squeeze out excess moisture.

Preheat oven at two hundred degrees Celsius. Use parchment paper for lining a baking tray.

Combine egg, cauliflower rice, ranch mix, and pepper in a bowl. Add the cheese. Mix well.

Take two tbsps. of the mixture and add them to the baking tray. Flatten with your hands. The thinner you can make the mixture, the crispier will be the crackers.

Bake for 10 minutes . Flip the crackers. Bake for 10 minutes .

Serve warm.

Nutrition: Calories: 29.6

Protein: 2.6g

Carbs: 1.1g

fat 2.6g

Fiber: 0.6g

231. Pork belly cracklins

Cooking Time: 1 hour and 35 minutes

Preparation Time: 10 minutes

Servings: 6

Ingredients

Three pounds of pork belly (with skin)

Two cups of water

Four tbsps. of Cajun seasoning

Directions:

Keep the pork belly in the refrigerator for forty minutes.

Cut the pork into cubes of three-fourth inch.

Fill a cast-iron pot with one-fourth portion of water. Add one tsp. of Cajun seasoning. Boil the water.

Add the cubes of pork belly.

Cook for twenty minutes.

Cover the pot once fat begins to pop and sizzle. Cook for fifteen minutes.

Drain the pork cracklins.

Sprinkle remaining seasoning from the top.

Serve immediately.

Nutrition: Calories: 210.3

Protein: 16.5g

Carbs: 1.5g

fat 16.6g

Fiber: 0.3g

232.   Lemon fat bombs

Cooking Time: Fifty minutes

Preparation Time: 10 minutes

Servings: 4

Ingredients

One cup of shredded coconut (dry)

One-fourth cup of coconut oil

Three tbsps. of erythritol sweetener (powdered)

Two tbsps. of lemon zest

One pinch of salt

Directions:

Add the coconut in a high power blender. Blend until creamy for fifteen minutes.

Add sweetener, coconut oil, salt, and lemon zest. Blend for two minutes.

Fill small muffin cups with the coconut mixture.

Chill in the refrigerator for thirty minutes.

Nutrition: Calories: 69.9

Protein: 0.5g

Carbs: 2.6g

fat 7.9g

Fiber: 1.1g

233.   Keto raspberry cake and white chocolate sauce

Servings: 5

Preparation time: 45 minutes

Cooking Time: 0 minutes

Ingredients:

For Cake

5 ounces cacao butter, melted

4 teaspoons of pure vanilla extract. You can replace with vanilla powder.

4 eggs

3 cup raspberries

2½ ounces grass-fed ghee

1 teaspoon baking powder

1 tablespoon of apple cider vinegar

1 cup green banana flour

¾ cup coconut cream

¾ cup of granulated sweetener

For the White chocolate sauce

4 ounces cacao butter

2 teaspoons pure vanilla extract

¾ cup of coconut cream

Pinch of salt

Directions:

Mix the butter and the sweetener together till they are completely mixed. You can make use mixer for this.

Pour in your grass-fed ghee into the mix, blend.

In a separate bowl, whisk the eggs together.

Take 2 ½ cups of the raspberries and slice them into halves.

Preheat your oven to 350 degrees F.

Get out a baking pan, and rub in the butter or spray it with cooking spray.

Pour in your mixed eggs to the butter and sweetener mixture. Mix well, until the sweetener disclosed wholly.

Pour in your banana flour and mix very well with a wooden spoon.

When mixed, mix in vanilla extract, apple cider, coconut cream, baking powder, and mix the mixture very well until batter form.

Spoon around the sliced berries lightly. Then, sprinkle just a little flour in your oiled or buttered baking pan

Hit the pan around, so the flour is absorbed by the oil or butter, dust out any extra flour.

Pour batter into the pan, and level it by smacking lightly on the counter.

Place in the oven, and bake for 45 minutes to an hour.

If you doubt its readiness, stick in a knife in the cake, and pull it out. If it comes out with any moistened, then it is not ready. We recommend you to run the cake test after 45 minutes. Not before.

When done take out, and leave it on a cake rack to cool.

For the sauce

Mix your cacao butter with 2 teaspoons pure vanilla extract.

Add coconut cream and beat the mixture very well.

Put in a pinch of salt to taste and beat again.

Chop up your remaining berries into tiny cubes and throw it in the mix.

Pour the mix on your cake and spread evenly.

Serve cold.

NUTRITION

Calories: 325 kcal

Total

fat 12g

Total Carbs: 3g

Protein: 40g

234. Keto chocolate chip cookies

Servings: 4

Preparation time: 40 minutes

Cooking Time: 0 minutes

Ingredients:

7 spoons of unsweetened coconut powder

7 tablespoons of Keto chocolate chips

5 tablespoons of butter

2 flat tablespoon of baking powder

2 eggs

2/3 confectioners swerve

1 1/3 cups of almond flour

A teaspoon of vanilla extract

Directions:

Preheat oven to 325˚.

Put in half of the chocolate chips and all the butter, and heat in the oven till it melts slightly.

Mix the melted chocolate and butter completely.

Crack and mix the eggs, and pour eggs in chocolate and butter mixture.

Mix in the vanilla extract, coconut powder, confectioners swerve, and almond flour. Mix well.

Add chocolate chip cookies. Remember to leave some chocolate chips to top the dough. Then, add baking powder, and mix until dough forms.

Spread out and cut out cookies, top with the rest of your chocolate chips.

Bake for 8 to 10 minutes. They will come out very soft.

Set them down and let them cool so they can harden. Enjoy.

NUTRITION

Calories: 287 kcal

Total

fat 19g

Total Carbs: 6.5g

Protein: 6.8g

235. Keto Beef and sausage balls

Servings: 3

Preparation time: 30 minutes

Cooking Time: 0 minutes

Ingredients:

MEAT

2 pounds of ground beef

2 pounds of ground sausage

2 eggs

½ cup of Keto mayonnaise

1/3 of cup ground pork rinds

½ cup of Parmesan cheese

Salt

Pepper

2 tablespoons of butter

3 tablespoons of oil

SAUCE

3 large diced onions

2 pounds of mushrooms sliced

5 sliced cloves of garlic

3 cups of beef broth

1 cup of sour cream

2 tablespoons of mustard

Worcestershire sauce

Salt

Pepper

Parsley

1 tablespoon of Arrowroot powder

Directions:

Put your meat, egg, and onions in a bowl. Mix with a spoon.

Put beef, parmesan, egg, mayonnaise, sausage, pork rind in a bowl.

Add salt and pepper to taste.

Heat oil or butter in a skillet.

Take the beef mix and mould into balls, place the balls in the oil and fry for 7-10 minutes.

When cooked, remove the balls from the pan and set aside.

Your skillet should still have oil, and so, you will put in your diced onions and fry till they brown a little.

Then, add the garlic and mushrooms, and sauté for 3 minutes. Then, add the broth.

Mix in mustard, sour cream and Worcestershire sauce well.

Boil for a minute or two then adds in the meatballs.

Add salt and pepper to your taste, let it simmer.

The arrowroot powder is to make the sauce thick.

If the sauce is already thick, you may ignore it.

Serve hot.

NUTRITION

Calories: 592 kcal

Total

fat 53.9g

Total Carbs: 1.3g

Protein: 25.4g

236. Keto coconut flake balls

Servings: 2

Preparation time: 15 minutes

Cooking Time: 0 minutes

Ingredients:

1 Vanilla Shortbread Collagen Protein Bar

1 tablespoon of lemon or coconut flavored FAT water In the absence, regular filter water is fine]

¼ teaspoon ground ginger

½ cup unsweetened coconut flakes,

¼ teaspoon ground turmeric

Directions:

Put protein bar, ginger, turmeric, and ¾ of the total flakes into a food processor, and process, until crumble. Avoid smoothing it.

Take out and add a spoon of water and roll till dough forms. If the spoonful is not enough, add a little more.

Roll into balls, and sprinkle the rest of your flakes on it or roll the balls in it.

Serve as it is or refrigerates it for a cold snack.

NUTRITION

Calories: 204 kcal

Total

fat 11g

Total Carbs: 4.2g

Protein: 1.5g

237. Keto chocolate Greek yoghurt cookies

Servings: 3

Preparation time: 1 hour

Cooking Time: 0 minutes

Ingredients:

3 eggs

1/8 teaspoon of tartar

5 tablespoons of softened Greek yoghurt

Directions:

Separate egg whites from the yolk and beat the whites until fluffy.

In the egg whites, pour the tartar, and mix well.

In the yolk, put in the Greek yoghurt, and mix well.

Combine both bowls' contents and mix thoroughly until thick.

With a spoon, line out scoops on the baking tray. Be sure to have parchment on the tray.

Lightly spread out the scoops, so they are like cookies. They will be very light, so apply no pressure.

Bake for 25-30 minutes, then take out and leave to cool for two hours.

NUTRITION

Calories: 287 kcal

Total fat 19g

Total Carbs: 6.5g

Protein: 6.8g

238. Keto coconut flavored ice cream

Servings: 4

Preparation time: 20 minutes

Cooking Time: 0 minutes

Ingredients:

4 cups of coconut milk

2/3 cup of xylitol or erythritol

¼ teaspoon of salt

2 teaspoons of vanilla extract

1 teaspoon of coconut extract

Directions:

Add the coconut milk in a bowl, with the sweetener, extracts, and salt. Stir well.

Pour this mixture in the ice cube trays, and put it in freezer.

When frozen, blend it at highest speed in a strong blender.

Freeze a little and consume same day.

NUTRITION

Calories: 244 kcal

Total

fat 48g

Total Carbs: 6g

Protein: 15g

239. Chocolate-coconut cookies

Servings: 4

Preparation time: 15 minutes

Cooking Time: 0 minutes

Ingredients:

2 eggs

½ cup of cocoa powder

½ cup of flour

½ cup of coconut oil

¼ cup of grated coconut

Stevia

Directions:

Preheat oven to 350 °F.

Crack eggs and separate whites and yolks mix well separately.

Add a pinch of salt to the yolks.

Heat oil in a skillet, and add cocoa, egg whites, stirring continuously, add in the salted yolks. Mix thoroughly. Then, add stevia to your taste.

Add in coconut flour and mix until dough forms.

On a clean flat surface, sprinkle grated coconut.

Roll the dough around in the coconut, so they mix well. Now, your dough is ready to be molded in cookies.

Bake for 15 minutes, let it cool to set.

NUTRITION

Calories: 260 kcal

Total

fat 26g

Total Carbs: 4.5g

Protein: 1g

240. Keto buffalo chicken meatballs

Servings: 3

Preparation time: 30 minutes

Cooking Time: 0 minutes

Ingredients:

1 pound of ground chicken

1 large

2/3 cup of hot sauce

½ cup of almond flour

½ teaspoon of salt

½ teaspoon of pepper

½ cup of melted butter

1 large chopped onion

1 teaspoon of minced garlic

Cooking spray or butter

Directions:

Combine meat, egg, and onions in a bowl, mix well with a spoon.

Pour in almond flour, garlic, salt, and pepper in, and mix well.

Preheat oven to 350°F, and prepare a baking tray by lining it with foil, then spray with cooking spray or rub butter thinly on it.

Mold the egg mixture into balls.

Set on the tray and bake for 18-20 minutes.

While it is done baking, place butter in microwave for few seconds to melt lightly.

Mix the melted butter and hot sauce in another bowl.

When the meatballs are slightly cooled, rub in this sauce.

Serve warm.

NUTRITION

Calories: 360 kcal

Total

fat 26g

Total Carbs: 4.5g

Protein: 1g

CHAPTER 18:

Desserts Recipes

241. British tartlets

Servings: 6

Cooking Time: 10 minutes

Preparation Time: 20 minutes

Ingredients:

For Crust: 2¼ C. almond flour ¼ C. powdered Swerve 5 tbsp. butter, melted ¼ tsp. sea salt

For Mascarpone Cream: 6 oz. mascarpone cheese, softened 2 tbsp. powdered Erythritol

1/3 C. heavy cream ¼ tsp. fresh lemon zest, grated 1 tsp. organic vanilla extract

For Garnishing: ½ C. fresh strawberries, hulled

Directions:

Preheat the oven to 350 0 F. Grease 6 (4-inch) tart pans. For crust: in a bowl, add all the ingredients and mix until well combined. Place the dough evenly into prepared tart pans and with your hands, press the mixture in the bottom and up sides. With a fork, prick the bottom of all crusts.

Bake for about 8-10 minutes.

Remove from the oven and place onto a wire rack to cool completely.

For the mascarpone cream: in a bowl, add mascarpone cheese, and Erythritol and with a mixer, beat on low speed for about 2 minutes. Slowly, add the heavy cream, beating continuously on low speed until well combined.

Now, beat on high speed for about 30-60 seconds or until thick.

Add the lemon zest, and vanilla extract and beat until well combined.

Transfer the mascarpone cream into a piping bag, fitted with a large star shaped tip and fill the tartlets.

Garnish with fresh strawberries and serve.

Nutrition:

Calories: 414

Carbohydrates: 10.8g

Protein: 12.5g

fat 35.7g

Sugar: 0.6g

Sodium: 188mg

Fiber: 4.8g

242. Sweet & tangy tart

Servings: 12,

Cooking Time: 25 minutes,

Preparation Time: 20 minutes

Ingredients:

For Lemon Curd:

3 organic eggs

10 tbsp. powdered Erythritol

6 tbsp. fresh lemon juice

2 tsp. fresh lemon zest, grated

2 tbsp. butter

For Crust:

1½ C. blanched almond flour ½ C. coconut flour 4 tbsp. powdered Erythritol 2 organic eggs

4 tbsp. cold unsalted butter

For Topping:

12 oz. fresh raspberries

Directions:

For lemon curd: in a small non-stick pan, add the eggs, and Erythritol and beat until well combined. Now, add the lemon juice, and zest and beat until well combined.

Place the pan over medium-low heat and cook for about 5-10 minutes or until mixture becomes thick, stirring continuously. Add the butter and stir until melted completely.

Remove from heat and transfer the curd into a bowl. With a cling film, cover the bowl and set aside for about 1 hour.

Then, refrigerate for about 2 hours. Preheat the oven to 350 0 F. Line the bottom of 2 (9-inch) greased tart pans with a removable bottom.

For crust: in a large bowl, add all the ingredients and mix until a dough ball comes together.

Divide the dough into 2 equal-sized portions.

Arrange 1 dough portion into each of the prepared tart pan and gently, press into the bottom to smooth the surface.

With a fork, prick the crust at many places.

Bake for about 15 minutes.

Remove the tart pans from oven and set aside to cool completely.

Gently and carefully, press each tart pan from the bottom to remove the sides.

Transfer each crust onto a platter.

Place the curd over each crust and with the back of a spoon, spread to smooth the surface.

Top each tart with fresh raspberries and serve.

Nutrition:

Calories: 198

Carbohydrates: 10.1g

Protein: 6.5g

fat 15g

Sugar: 1.6g

Sodium: 73mg

Fiber: 5.4g

243. Flour less Chocolate Cake

Servings: 8

Cooking Time: 15 minutes

Preparation Time: 28 minutes

Ingredients:

7 oz. 70% dark chocolate

chopped finely ½ C. olive oil

1 C. granulated Erythritol

5 large organic eggs

1 tsp. organic vanilla extract

4 tbsp. cacao powder

1 tsp. espresso powder

¼ tsp. salt

Directions:

Preheat the oven to 350 0 F. and lightly grease Line the bottom of a lightly greased 9-inch cake pan with parchment paper.

In a microwave-safe bowl, add the chocolate and oil and microwave for about 2 minutes, stirring after every 30 seconds.

Remove from the microwave and mix until smooth. Set aside to cool for about 2 of minutes.

Add the Erythritol and beat until well combined. Add the eggs, one at a time, beating well after each addition.

Add the vanilla extract and mix well. In another bowl, add the cocoa powder, espresso powder and salt and mix well. Add the cacao powder mixture into the chocolate mixture and mix until just combined.

Place the mixture into the prepared cake pan evenly. Bake for about 25-28 minutes or until a skewer inserted in the center of comes out clean.

Remove from the oven and place the pan onto a wire rack to cool for about 10-15 minutes.

Carefully invert the cake and place onto the wire rack to cool completely before slicing.

Cut into desired-sized slices and serve.

Nutrition: Calories: 326

Carbohydrates: 8.2g

Protein: 7.8g

fat 29.4g

Sugar: 0.3g

Sodium: 126mg

Fiber: 4.1g

244. Melt-in-Moth Lava Cake

Servings: 2

Cooking Time: 9 minutes

Preparation Time: 15 minutes

Ingredients:

2 oz. 70% dark chocolate 2 oz. unsalted butter 2 organic eggs

2 tbsp. powdered Erythritol plus more for dusting 1 tbsp. almond flour 6 fresh raspberries

Directions:

Preheat the oven to 350 0 F. Grease 2 ramekins.

In a microwave-safe bowl, add the chocolate and butter and microwave on High for about 2 minutes or until melted, stirring after every 30 seconds.

Remove from the microwave and stir until smooth.

Place the eggs in a bowl and with a wire whisk, beat well. Add the chocolate mixture, Erythritol and almond flour and mix until well combined. Divide the mixture into the prepared ramekins evenly.

Bake for about 9 minutes or until the top is set.

Remove from oven and set aside for about 1-2 minutes.

Carefully, invert the cakes onto the serving plates and dust with extra powdered Erythritol. Serve with a garnishing of the strawberries.

Nutrition:

Calories: 436 Carbohydrates: 11g

Protein: 10.4g fat 25.2g

Sugar: 1.4g Sodium: 232mg Fiber: 6.1g

245. British tartlets

Servings: 6

Cooking Time: 10 minutes

Preparation Time: 20 minutes

Ingredients:

For Crust: 2¼ C. almond flour ¼ C. powdered Swerve 5 tbsp. butter, melted ¼ tsp. sea salt

For Mascarpone Cream: 6 oz. mascarpone cheese, softened 2 tbsp. powdered Erythritol

1/3 C. heavy cream ¼ tsp. fresh lemon zest, grated 1 tsp. organic vanilla extract

For Garnishing: ½ C. fresh strawberries, hulled

Directions: Preheat the oven to 350 0 F.

Grease 6 (4-inch) tart pans. For crust: in a bowl, add all the ingredients and mix until well combined. Place the dough evenly into prepared tart pans and with your hands, press the mixture in the bottom and up sides.

With a fork, prick the bottom of all crusts.

Bake for about 8-10 minutes. Remove from the oven and place onto a wire rack to cool completely. For the mascarpone cream: in a bowl, add mascarpone cheese, and Erythritol and with a mixer, beat on low speed for about 2 minutes.

Slowly, add the heavy cream, beating continuously on low speed until well combined. Now, beat on high speed for about 30-60 seconds or until thick.

Add the lemon zest, and vanilla extract and beat until well combined. Transfer the mascarpone cream into a piping bag, fitted with a large star shaped tip and fill the tartlets.

Garnish with fresh strawberries and serve.

Nutrition:

Calories: 414 Carbohydrates: 10.8g

Protein: 12.5g fat 35.7g

Sugar: 0.6g Sodium: 188mg

Fiber: 4.8g

246. Sweet & tangy tart

Servings: 12

Cooking Time: 25 minutes

Preparation Time: 20 minutes

Ingredients:

For Lemon Curd:

3 organic eggs

10 tbsp. powdered Erythritol

6 tbsp. fresh lemon juice

2 tsp. fresh lemon zest, grated

2 tbsp. butter

For Crust:

1½ C. blanched almond flour

½ C. coconut flour

4 tbsp. powdered Erythritol

2 organic eggs

4 tbsp. cold unsalted butter

For Topping:

12 oz. fresh raspberries

Directions:

For lemon curd: in a small non-stick pan, add the eggs, and Erythritol and beat until well combined.

Now, add the lemon juice, and zest and beat until well combined.

Place the pan over medium-low heat and cook for about 5-10 minutes or until mixture becomes thick, stirring continuously.

Add the butter and stir until melted completely.

Remove from heat and transfer the curd into a bowl.

With a cling film, cover the bowl and set aside for about 1 hour.

Then, refrigerate for about 2 hours.

Preheat the oven to 350 0 F. Line the bottom of 2 (9-inch) greased tart pans with a removable bottom.

For crust: in a large bowl, add all the ingredients and mix until a dough ball comes together.

Divide the dough into 2 equal-sized portions.

Arrange 1 dough portion into each of the prepared tart pan and gently, press into the bottom to smooth the surface.

With a fork, prick the crust at many places.

Bake for about 15 minutes.

Remove the tart pans from oven and set aside to cool completely.

Gently and carefully, press each tart pan from the bottom to remove the sides.

Transfer each crust onto a platter.

Place the curd over each crust and with the back of a spoon, spread to smooth the surface. Top each tart with fresh raspberries and serve.

Nutrition:

Calories: 198 Carbohydrates: 10.1g

Protein: 6.5g fat 15g Sugar: 1.6g

Sodium: 73mg Fiber: 5.4g

247. Light greek yogurt cheesecake

Servings: 8

Cooking Time: 35 minutes

Preparation Time: 15 minutes

Ingredients:

2½ C. plain Greek yogurt

6-8 drops of liquid stevia

3 organic egg whites

1/3 C. cacao powder

¼ C. arrowroot starch

1 tsp. organic vanilla extract

Pinch of sea salt

Directions:

Preheat the oven to 35 0 F. Grease a 9-inch cake pan.

In a large bowl, add all ingredients and mix until well combined. Place the mixture into the prepared pan evenly.

Bake for about 30-35 minutes.

Remove from oven and let it cool completely. Refrigerate to chill for about 3-4 hours or until set completely.

Cut into 8 equal sized slices and serve.

Nutrition:

Calories: 85

Carbohydrates: 10g

Protein: 6.4g

fat 1.6g

Sugar: 5g

Sodium: 97mg

Fiber: 2g

248. Swiss roll cake

Servings: 10

Cooking Time: 10 minutes

Preparation Time: 20 minutes

Ingredients:

For Cake:

1 C. almond flour

½ C. powdered Swerve

¼ C. matcha powder

¼ C. psyllium husk powder

1 tsp. organic baking powder

½ tsp. salt

3 large organic eggs

½ C. heavy whipping cream

4 tbsp. butter, melted

1 tsp. organic vanilla extract

For Filling:

3-4 tbsp. water

1 packet unflavored gelatin

2 C. heavy whipping cream

2 tsp. organic vanilla extract

¼ C. powdered Swerve

Directions:

Preheat oven to 350 0 F. Line a baking sheet with parchment paper.

For cake: in a bowl, add almond flour, Swerve, matcha powder, psyllium husk, baking powder and salt and mix well.

Now, sift the flour mixture into a second bowl.

In a third bowl, add remaining ingredients and beat until well combined.

Add the egg mixture into the bowl of flour mixture and mix until a very thick dough forms.

Place the dough onto prepared baking sheet and roll into an even rectangle.

Bake for about 10 minutes.

Remove from oven and put onto a wire rack to cool for about 4-5 minutes.

Gently, roll the warm cake with the help of parchment paper.

Set aside to cool completely.

For filling: in a microwave-safe bowl, add the water and sprinkle with the gelatin. Set aside for about 5 minutes.

Now, microwave for about 15-20 seconds. Remove from microwave and beat the gelatin mixture until smooth.

Place gelatin mixture and remaining ingredients in bowl of the stand mixer and beat until cream becomes stiff. Spread the whipped cream over cooled cake evenly.

Carefully and gently, roll the cake and freezer for about 10 minutes before slicing.

Cut into desired sized slices and serve.

Nutrition:

Calories: 249

Carbohydrates: 7.1g

Protein: 5.6g

fat 22.8g

Sugar: 0.7g

Sodium: 183mg

Fiber: 4g

249. Kale chips

Servings: 4

Preparation Time: 10 min

Cooking Time: 12 minutes

Ingredients:

Kale: 1 bunch

Chili powder: 1 teaspoon

Garlic powder: ½ teaspoon

Ground cumin: ½ teaspoon

Sea salt: ½ teaspoon

Pepper: ¼ teaspoon

Cayenne: 1/8 teaspoon

Avocado oil: ¼ cup

Nutritional yeast: ¼ cup

Directions:

1.   Cut the kale into pieces and wash and dry.

Mix together the chili powder, cumin, garlic powder, pepper, cayenne and salt.

Toss together the kale, oil, spice mix and yeast in a bowl.

Spread the kale on two baking sheets and bake for 10 minutes.

Turn off the oven and leave inside for 2-5 minutes.

Nutrition:

108 Cal,

14.54 g total fat,

7.68 g carbs,

2.24 g fiber,

3.6 g protein.

250. Eggplant bruschetta

These are scrumptious low-carb appetizers.

Servings: 4

Preparation Time: 10 min

Cooking Time: 5-7 minutes

Ingredients:

Eggplant -sliced into circles - 1

Salt: ½ teaspoon

Olive oil: 2 tablespoon

Pepper: to taste

Topping:

Fresh tomatoes -diced: 2 cups

Basil -chopped: 2 tablespoon

Garlic cloves -minced - 2

Olive oil: 1 tablespoon

Salt and pepper to taste

Directions:

Mix together all the topping ingredients in a bowl.

Season the eggplant with salt and leave aside for 30 minutes.

Grill the eggplant for 5-7 minutes per side on a preheated grill.

Brush oil on the eggplant and season with pepper.

Spoon the topping over the eggplant slices and enjoy.

Nutrition:

71 Cal,

5 g total fat,

206 mg sodium,

4 g net carbs,

2 g fiber,

1g protein.

251. Mushroom chips

Servings: 4

Preparation Time: 10 min

Cooking Time: 45-60 minutes

Ingredients:

Portobello mushrooms -slice thinly: 10.6 oz.

Coconut oil: 4 tablespoon

Salt: ½ teaspoon

Black pepper -ground: just a dash

Directions:

Place the mushrooms on a non-stick baking sheet and brush the oil on it.

Sprinkle with salt and pepper.

Bake for 45-60 minutes in an oven preheated to 300 degrees Fahrenheit, flipping thrice in between.

Nutrition:

169 Cal,

15.5 g total fat,

5.8 g carbs,

2 g fiber,

3.2 g protein.

252. Strawberry Ice cream

Servings: 5

Preparation Time: 10 min

Cooking Time: 2 min

Ingredients:

Full fat coconut milk: 1 can

Water: 1 cup

Glucomannan powder: 1 teaspoon

Strawberries: 1 cup

Vanilla extract: 1 teaspoon

Stevia drops: to taste

Directions:

Combine the water and glucomannan powder in a saucepan over low flame and stir until it dissolves and a gel is formed.

Combine all the ingredients including the gel in a blender and blend until smooth.

Chill for an hour and then transfer into an ice cream maker.

Nutrition:

141 Cal,

13 g total fat,

3 g net carbs,

1 g fiber,

1 g protein.

253. Pumpkin spice brownies

Servings: 12

Preparation Time: 10 min

Cooking Time: 40 min

Ingredients:

Canned pumpkin puree: 1 cup

Coconut flour: ¼ cup

Tahini: ½ cup

Swerve - 1/4 cup

Pumpkin pie spice: 1 tablespoon

Apple cider vinegar: 1 tablespoon

Baking powder: 1 teaspoon

Vanilla extract: 1 teaspoon

Directions:

Mix together all the dry ingredients in one bowl and all the wet ingredients in another bowl.

Combine together both the dry and wet ingredients and mix well.

Spread the mixture into a greased brownie pan.

Bake for 40 minutes in an oven preheated to 350 degrees Fahrenheit.

Nutrition:

79 Cal,

5.6 g total fat,

1.8 g net carbs,

2.5 g fiber,

3.2 g protein.

254. Pecan & maple fudge

Servings: 16

Preparation Time: 15 min

Ingredients:

Butter:

Pecans: 3 cups

Vanilla powder: ½ teaspoon

Cinnamon -ground: ½ teaspoon

Sugar-free maple extract: 1 teaspoon

Salt: just a pinch

Fudge:

Powdered erythritol - ¼ cup

Coconut oil: ½ cup

Pecans -chopped: 1 ¼ cup

Pecan halves - 16

Directions:

Combine all the butter ingredients in a food processor and process until smooth.

Add in the coconut oil and erythritol and pulse again.

Transfer into a pan lined with parchment paper.

Spread with a spatula and mix in the chopped pecans.

Sprinkle the pecan halves on top.

Refrigerate for 2 hours till set and then cut into pieces.

Nutrition:

247 Cal,

26 g total fat,

5.4 g sat. fat,

4.2 g carbs,

2.8 g fiber,

2.6 g protein.

255. Coconut cupcakes

Servings: 7

Preparation Time: 10 min

Ingredients:

Vanilla flavored protein powder: 4 ¼ oz.

Coconut flakes -unsweetened: 3 oz.

Coconut milk -unsweetened: 0.84 cup

Coconut oil: 4 tablespoon

Psyllium husk: 2 tablespoon

Dark chocolate - cocoa: ¾ oz.

Directions:

Mix together the protein powder, psyllium and coconut flakes.

Mix in the coconut oil and coconut milk.

Pour the mixture into cupcake forms.

Melt the chocolate and spread it over.

Freeze for 30 minutes.

Sprinkle the pecan halves on top.

Refrigerate for 2 hours till set and then cut into pieces.

Nutrition:

371 Cal,

30.7 g total fat,

10.1 g carbs,

5.85 g fiber,

17.15 g protein.

256. Rutabaga cakes

Servings: 12

Preparation Time:10 min

Cooking Time:40 min

Ingredients:

Rutabagas -sliced thinly - 2

Butter -melted: ½ stick

Fresh thyme -chopped: 2 tablespoons

Salt: 2 teaspoons

Directions:

Heat the butter in a saucepan and add the thyme to it, stirring continuously for 2 minutes.

Place the rutabaga slices in a bowl and pour the buttery mixture over it.

Layer the rutabaga slices in muffin tins and drizzle the rest of the butter over.

Using a foil, cover the muffin tin and bake in an oven preheated to 350 degrees Fahrenheit for 25-30 minutes.

Nutrition:

46 Cal,

3.9 g total fat,

2.1 g net carbs,

0.4 g protein.

257. Jalapeno poppers

Servings: 8

Preparation Time:10 min

Cooking Time:25 min

Ingredients:

Jalapeno pepper: 1 lb.

Garlic powder: 1 teaspoon

Scallions -sliced finely, green tops only- 1 bunch

Paprika: to taste

Cream cheese -softened: 8 oz.

Yellow Cheddar cheese -shredded: 1 cup

Directions:

Slice the jalapeno pepper, leaving the stem intact.

Scoop out the seeds.

For the stuffing, mix together all the rest of the ingredients in a bowl and stuff it into the jalapenos.

Bake in an oven preheated to 350 degrees Fahrenheit for 25 minutes.

Nutrition:

179 Cal,

14.7 g total fat –

8.5 g sat. fat,

46.1 mg chol.,

184.4 mg sodium,

7 g carbs,

2.2 g fiber,

6.2 g protein.

258. Roasted radish chips

Servings: 4

Preparation Time:10 min

Cooking Time:15 min

Ingredients:

Fresh radish -chopped thinly into rounds: 16 oz.

Sea salt: ½ teaspoon

Pepper: ½ teaspoon

Coconut oil: 2 tablespoon

Directions:

Toss together all the ingredients and spread on baking sheets with any overlap.

Bake in an oven preheated to 400 degrees Fahrenheit for another 12-15 minutes.

Nutrition:

70 Cal,

7.1 g total fat -

6 g sat. fat,

0 mg chol.,

304 mg sodium,

2.2 g carbs,

1 g fiber,

0.4 g protein.

259. Raspberry candies

Servings: 6

Preparation Time:10 min

Ingredients:

Cream cheese -room temperature: 4 oz.

Butter: 4 tablespoon

Coconut oil: ¼ cup

Liquid stevia: 2 teaspoon

Raspberries: 12

Lime juice: 1 tablespoon

Directions:

Melt the coconut oil and butter and then stir in the cream cheese.

Mix in the rest of the ingredients and pour the mixture into a silicon heart-shaped candy tray.

Leave to freeze for ½ an hour.

Nutrition:

221 Cal,

22 g total fat,

5 g carbs,

2 g fiber,

0 g protein.

260. Choco brownies

Servings: 20

Preparation Time:10 min

Cooking Time: 15 min

Ingredients:

Cream cheese -room temperature: 1/3 cup

Butter: 2 tablespoon

Eggs: 3

Cocoa powder -unsweetened: 4 tablespoon

Almond flour: 4 tablespoon

Coconut flour: 4 tablespoon

Stevia: 4 tablespoon

Vanilla extract: 1 teaspoon

Baking powder: ¼ teaspoon

Coconut milk: ¼ cup

Directions:

Combine all the ingredients in a bowl and mix well until smooth.

Pour the mixture into a 9x13 inch pan greased with coconut oil.

Bake for 15 minutes in an oven preheated to 350 degrees Fahrenheit.

Leave to cool and chop into 20 pieces.

Nutrition:

57 Cal,

5 g total fat,

3 mg chol.,

39 mg sodium,

2 g carbs,

1 g fiber,

2 g protein.

261. Pumpkin butter cookies

Servings: 27

Preparation Time: 15 min

Cooking Time: 20 min

Ingredients:

Almond flour: 2 cups

Organic pumpkin: ½ cup

Egg: 1

Butter: ½ cup

Pure vanilla extract: 1 teaspoon

Baking powder: ½ teaspoon

Pumpkin pie spice: ½ teaspoon

Liquid stevia: 1 teaspoon

Directions:

Combine all the ingredients in a bowl and mix well.

Roll portions of the mixture, making 27 balls and place on a sil-eco baking mat.

Press down the dough lightly using a fork.

Bake for 20-23 minutes in an oven preheated to 300 degrees Fahrenheit.

Nutrition:

82 Cal,

8 g total fat,

16 mg chol.,

34 mg sodium,

2 g carbs, 1 g fiber,

2 g protein.

262. Tantalizing apple pie bites

Serving: 4

Preparation Time: 20 minutes

Cooking Time: 0 minutes

Ingredients

1 cup chopped walnuts

½ a cup of coconut oil

¼ cup of ground flaxseed

½ ounce of frozen dried apples

1 teaspoon of vanillaextract

1 teaspoon of cinnamon

Liquid Stevia

Directions

Melt the coconut oil until it is liquid

Take your blender and add walnuts, coconut oil, and process well

Add flaxseeds, vanilla, and Stevia

Keep processing until a fine mixture form

Stop and add crumbled dried apples

Process until your desired texture appears

Portion the mixture amongst muffin molds and allow them to chill

Enjoy!

Nutrition

Calories: 194

fat 19g

Carbs: 2g

Protein: 2.3g

263. Vegan compliant protein balls

Serving: 8

Preparation Time: 20 minutes

Cooking Time: 0 minutes

Ingredients

1 cup of creamed coconut

2 scoops of Vega Sport Chocolate Protein -or any protein powder of your preference

¼ cup of ground flax seed

½ a teaspoon of vanillaextract

½ a teaspoon of mint extract

1-2 tablespoon of cocoa powder

Directions

Take a large sized bowl and melt the creamed coconut

Add the vanilla extract and stir well

Stir in flax seed, protein powder and knead until the fine dough forms

Form 24 balls and allow the balls to chill for 10-15 minutes

Roll them up in some cocoa powder if you prefer and serve!

Nutrition

Calories: 260

fat 20g

Carbs: 3g

Protein: 10g

264. The keto lovers "magical" grain free granola

Serving: 10

Preparation Time: 10 minutes

Cooking Time: 75 minutes

Ingredients

½ a cup of raw sunflower seeds

½ a cup of raw hemp hearts

½ a cup of flaxseeds

¼ cup of chia seeds

2 tablespoon of Psyllium Husk powder

1 tablespoon of cinnamon

Stevia

½ a teaspoon of baking powder

½ a teaspoon of salt

1 cup of water

Directions

Pre-heat your oven to 300 degrees Fahrenheit

Line up a baking sheet with parchment paper

Take your food processor and grind all the seeds

Add the dry ingredients and mix well

Stir in water until fully incorporated

Allow the mixture to sit for a while until it thickens up

Spread the mixture evenly on top of your baking sheet -giving a thickness of about ¼ inch

Bake for 45 minutes

Break apart the granola and keep baking for another 30 minutes until the pieces are crunchy

Remove and allow them to cool

Enjoy!

Nutrition

Calories: 292

fat 25g

Carbs: 12g

Protein: 8g

265. Ultimate peanut butter cookies

Cooking Time: 15 minutes

Preparation Time: 10 minutes

Servings 12

Ingredients

1 ¼ cups peanut butter

1 cup granulated monk fruit

2 tablespoons flaxseed meal

2 tablespoons ground chia seeds

Directions

Start by preheating your oven to 360 degrees F. Then, coat a baking pan with parchment paper.

In a mixing bowl, thoroughly combine all ingredients until everything is well incorporated.

Shape the mixture into bite-sized balls. Press each ball into a cookie shape using a fork.

Bake in the preheated oven for 9 minutes, or until lightly golden at the edges. Place your cookies on wire racks before serving. Enjoy!

Nutrition:

143 Calories

9.3g Fat

7.4g Carbs

6.8g Protein

2.4g Fiber

266. Chocolate almond cookies

Cooking Time: 15 minutes

Preparation Time: 10 minutes

Servings 12

Ingredients

1 cup almond flour

1/2 cup almond butter

1/2 cup sesame butter

1/2 cup granulated Erythritol

2 tablespoons chia seeds, ground

1 teaspoon vanilla extract

1/4 teaspoon grated nutmeg

1/4 cup cocoa, unsweetened

Directions

Start by preheating your oven to 360 degrees F. Prepare a silicone baking sheet.

Then, combine all ingredients with a hand mixer.

Using a cookie scoop or your hands, form the dough into small balls. Arrange them on the prepared baking sheet.

Press lightly using a spoon. Bake in the preheated oven for about 10 minutes, or until lightly golden at the edges. Bon appétit!

Nutrition:

178 Calories 15.4g Fat

6.4g Carbs 6.1g Protein

3.2g Fiber

267. Cinnamon brownie bars

Cooking Time: 1 hour 5 minutes

Preparation Time: 10 minutes

Servings 12

Ingredients

1/2 cup almonds, ground

1/2 cup walnuts, ground

1 cup granulated monk fruit

1/3 cup cocoa powder, unsweetened

1 teaspoon ground cinnamon

1/2 teaspoon vanilla extract

2 tablespoons coconut oil

A pinch of sea salt

Directions

Mix all ingredients until everything is well incorporated. Scrape the batter into a lightly greased baking sheet.

Let it sit in your freezer for 1 hour.

Cut into squares and serve well chilled. Enjoy!

Nutrition:

71 Calories

6.7g Fat

2.9g Carbs

1.7g Protein

1.5g Fiber

268. Easy raspberry jam

Cooking Time: 15 minutes

Preparation Time: 10 minutes

Servings 5

Ingredients

1 cup raspberries, fresh or frozen

4 tablespoons chia seeds, ground

1/4 teaspoon ground cloves

1 teaspoon vanilla paste

1/3 cup water

1 teaspoon orange juice

1 teaspoon orange zest

2 tablespoons powdered monk fruit

Directions

Combine all ingredients in the bowl of your food processor. Puree the mixture to the desired consistency.

Taste and adjust for sweetness.

Place your jam in a jar and store in the refrigerator.

Nutrition:

71 Calories

3.6g Fat

7.3g Carbs

2.2g Protein

5.5g Fiber

269. Raspberry and almond swirl cheesecake

Cooking Time: 3 hours 10 minutes

Preparation Time: 10 minutes

Servings 8

Ingredients

Crust:

1 cup blanched almond flour

1 tablespoon coconut oil

1/8 teaspoon grated nutmeg

1/4 teaspoon kosher salt

1/2 teaspoon liquid stevia

Cheesecake:

1 cup blanched almonds, soaked in hot water for 2 hours

1/4 cup almond milk

1/2 cup coconut oil, melted

1 teaspoon vanilla paste

2 tablespoons fresh lime juice

Filling:

1 cup keto raspberry jam, preferably homemade

Directions

In your food processor, pulse together all ingredients for the crust. Press the almond crust into a small baking pan lined with parchment paper. Set aside.

Drain and rinse the soaked almonds

pulse your almonds in a food processor until a ball form.

Stir in the remaining ingredients for the cheesecake and blend again until creamy and smooth.

Pour the mixture over the prepared crust and let it sit in your freezer for about 3 hours or until set.

Top your cheesecake with small spoonsful of raspberry jam

use a toothpick to create swirl patterns on top of the cheesecake. Enjoy!

Nutrition:

216 Calories

21.6g Fat

4.9g Carbs

2.9g Protein

2.5g Fiber

270. Perfect peppermint fudge

Cooking Time: 1 hour 10 minutes

Preparation Time: 10 minutes

Servings 6

Ingredients

1/2 cup coconut oil, melted

1/3 cup sugar-free chocolate chips, melted

1/4 cup hemp hearts, soaked overnight and rinsed

1 teaspoon peppermint extract

1/8 teaspoon kosher salt

1/8 teaspoon nutmeg, preferably freshly grated

Directions

Pulse all ingredients in your food processor until smooth and uniform.

Spoon the prepared mixture into a baking pan. Place you fudge in the refrigerator for 1 hour.

Allow your fudge to cool completely before cutting into 1-inch squares. Bon appétit!

Nutrition:

191 Calories

20.2g Fat

3.6g Carbs

1g Protein

0.2g Fiber

271.   Chewy chocolate and peanut butter bars

Cooking Time: 25 minutes

Preparation Time: 10 minutes

Servings 8

Ingredients

Base Layer:

1/2 cup peanut butter

2 tablespoons ground almonds

2 tablespoons granulated monk fruit

Top Layer:

1/4 cup peanut butter

1/4 cup sesame butter

2 tablespoons cocoa powder, unsweetened

1 tablespoon granulated monk fruit

2 tablespoons coconut flour

Directions

Mix all ingredients for the base layer in a bowl

in a separate bowl, mix the ingredients for the top layer. Mix to combine well.

Line a baking pan with parchment paper. Spread the base layer on the parchment paper

spread the top layer on it and transfer to the preheated oven.

Bake for 20 to 22 minutes at 350 degrees F. Place on wire racks before cutting and serving. Bon appétit!

Nutrition:

237 Calories

19.9g Fat

7.3g Carbs

7.6g Protein

2.8g Fiber

272.   Festive butterscotch blondies

Cooking Time: 25 minutes

Preparation Time: 10 minutes

Servings 12

Ingredients

1 tablespoon flaxseed meal

4 tablespoons almond milk

1 cup almond butter

1/4 cup granulated monk fruit

1/4 teaspoon grated nutmeg

1 teaspoon vanilla extract

1 teaspoon baking powder

A pinch of salt

1/2 cup vegan butterscotch chips

Directions

Start by preheating your oven to 350 degrees F

now, line a baking dish with parchment paper and set aside.

In a mixing bowl, thoroughly combine the flaxseed meal, almond milk, almond butter, granulated monk fruit, nutmeg, vanilla, baking powder, and salt

mix until everything is well incorporated. Fold in the butterscotch chips.

Press the batter into the prepared baking dish

press it using a wide spatula or your hands.

Bake in the preheated oven for about 18 minutes or until it is lightly golden

transfer to a cooling rack before slicing and serving. Enjoy!

Nutrition:

162 Calories

13.2g Fat

6.2g Carbs

5.1g Protein

3g Fiber

273. Blackberry jam sandwich cookies

Cooking Time: 2 hours 40 minutes

Preparation Time: 10 minutes

Servings 10

Ingredients

Filling:

16 ounces fresh blackberries

1/4 cup granulated Swerve

1/8 teaspoon xanthan gum

Cookies:

3 cups unsweetened coconut, shredded

4 tablespoons monk fruit sweetener

1/3 cup coconut milk

1/2 teaspoon vanilla extract

Directions

Place the blackberries and granulated Swerve in your slow cooker. Cook for 2 hours 30 minutes on low heat.Afterwards, stir in the xanthan gum to thicken the jam. Meanwhile, pulse all ingredients for the cookies until everything is well combined. Now, roll the batter until 1/4-thick. Place on a parchment paper-lined baking sheet and chill until firm or at least 1 hour. Using a 2-inch fluted round cutter, cut out the cookies. Spread half the cookies with 1/2 teaspoon of jam each assemble the cookie sandwiches with the rest of the cookies. Bon appétit!

Nutrition:

119 Calories 9.8g Fat 7.2g Carbs

1.6g Protein 4.6g Fiber

274. Coconut carrot cake squares

Cooking Time: 40 minutes

Preparation Time: 10 minutes

Servings 8

Ingredients

Carrot Cake Base:

1 cup coconut flour

1 cup water

4 tablespoons applesauce, unsweetened

1/4 teaspoon ground cloves

1 teaspoon vanilla extract

1 teaspoon ground cinnamon

1/4 cup granulated monk fruit

1 large carrot, shredded

Topping:

1/4 cup shredded coconut

Directions

Mix all ingredients for the carrot cake base until well combined.

Press the mixture into a parchment-lined baking pan. Place in your refrigerator for 30 minutes.

Scatter the shredded coconut over the top and cut into squares. Enjoy!

Nutrition:

53 Calories 4.2g Fat

3.9g Carbs 0.7g Protein

1.6g Fiber

275. The best avocado cupcakes ever

Cooking Time: 30 minutes

Preparation Time: 10 minutes

Servings 12

Ingredients

1/2 cup ripe avocado, mashed

1/3 cup coconut oil

1 cup hot water

1 tablespoon instant coffee

1 cup coconut flour

1 cup cocoa powder, unsweetened

8 ounces erythritol

1 teaspoon baking soda

1/2 teaspoon vanilla extract

1/4 teaspoon ground cardamom

1/4 teaspoon kosher salt

Directions

Start by preheating your oven to 355 degrees F. Prepare the cupcake molds and set aside. In a mixing bowl, thoroughly combine the avocado with the coconut oil. Dissolve the instant coffee in hot water and stir into the avocado mixture. Stir in the other ingredients. Divide the batter between the cupcake molds. Bake in the preheated oven for 20 to 25 minutes. Transfer to a wire rack to cool completely. Bon appétit!

Nutrition:

107 Calories 10.5g Fat 6.2g Carbs

1.7g Protein 3.4g Fiber

276. Key lime mini cheesecakes

Cooking Time: 30 minutes

Preparation Time: 10 minutes

Servings 12

Ingredients

Crust:

1 cup almond meal

4 tablespoons coconut oil

A pinch of salt

A pinch of freshly grated nutmeg

Cheesecake:

1 cup cashews, soaked in hot water for 2 hours

1/4 cup almond milk

1/2 cup coconut oil, melted

1 tablespoon fresh key lime juice

1 teaspoon key lime zest, grated

1 teaspoon vanilla paste

Directions

Line a muffin tin with cupcake liners and set aside.

In your food processor, pulse together all ingredients for the crust. Press the crust into the bottom of a muffin tin.

Bake the crusts at 350 degrees F for about 5 minutes or until it is slightly brown and crispy.

Drain and rinse the soaked cashews

pulse in a food processor until a ball forms. Stir in the remaining ingredients for the cheesecake and blend until creamy.

Pour the mixture over the prepared crust. Let them cool in the refrigerator overnight. Bon appétit!

Nutrition:

167 Calories

17.5g Fat

2.9g Carbs

1.7g Protein

0.3g Fiber

277. Home-style chocolate bar

Cooking Time: 30 minutes

Preparation Time: 10 minutes

Servings 4

Ingredients

6 tablespoons coconut oil

2 ounces sugar-free unsweetened baker's chocolate

2 tablespoons tofu, pureed

4 tablespoons powdered erythritol

1/2 teaspoon vanilla extract

1/4 teaspoon grated nutmeg

1/4 teaspoon ground cloves

1/8 teaspoon coarse sea salt

Directions

Microwave the coconut oil and chocolate and stir well. Stir in the tofu and powdered erythritol.

Add the remaining ingredients and stir until everything is well combined. Pour the chocolate mixture into a chocolate mold.

Freeze for 1 to 2 hours and serve!

Nutrition:

190 Calories

20.8g Fat

3.3g Carbs

0.7g Protein

0.4g Fiber

278. Chocolate avocado pudding

Cooking Time: 10 minutes + chilling time

Preparation Time: 10 minutes

Servings 4

Ingredients

1 ½ cups canned full-fat coconut milk

1/2 cup cacao powder, unsweetened

1 teaspoon pure vanilla extract

1/4 teaspoon grated nutmeg

1/2 teaspoon ground cinnamon

1/8 teaspoon kosher salt

1 avocado, peeled, pitted and mashed

1/2 cup powdered monk fruit

Directions

Heat the coconut milk and cacao powder in a saucepan over low heat stir to combine well.

Remove from the heat and cool slightly. Transfer the mixture to a blender and stir in the remaining ingredients.

Blend until creamy and uniform. Place in your refrigerator for 2 to 3 hours. Serve well-chilled!

Nutrition:

226 Calories

21.1g Fat

7.7g Carbs

4.7g Protein

5g Fiber

279. Old-fashioned walnut cookies

Cooking Time: 10 minutes + chilling time

Preparation Time: 10 minutes

Servings 8

Ingredients

1/2 cup almond meal

1/2 cup coconut flour

2 cups no-sugar dairy-free chocolate spread

1/2 cup monk fruit

1/2 teaspoon vanilla extract

1/2 teaspoon ground cinnamon

1/4 teaspoon ground cardamom

2 tablespoon almond milk

1 cup walnuts, finely chopped

Directions

Coat a cookie sheet with parchment paper

set aside.

Thoroughly combine all ingredients, except for the walnuts, in a mixing bowl. Roll the mixture into bite-sized balls.

Arrange these balls on the prepared cookie sheet.

In a shallow dish, place the walnuts. Cover the prepared cookies with the chopped walnuts and press them into a cookie shape

place in your refrigerator until firm. Bon appétit!

Nutrition:

200 Calories

18g Fat

7.8g Carbs

6.6g Protein

4.9g Fiber

CHAPTER 19:

Keto Diet Shopping List

Keto Shopping List for Saving Money and Time Without Wasting Food

Seafood

Seafood means fish like sardines, mackerel, and wild salmon. It's also a good idea to add some shrimp, tuna, mussels, and crab into your diet. This is going to be a tad expensive, but worth it in the long run. What's the common denominator in all these food items? The secret is omega-3 fatty acids, which are credited for lots of health benefits. You want to add food rich in omega-3 fatty acids in your diet.

Low-carb Vegetables

Not all vegetables are good for you when it comes to the Ketogenic Diet. The vegetable choices should be limited to those with low carbohydrate counts. Pack up your cart with items like spinach, eggplant, arugula, broccoli, and cauliflower. You can also put in bell peppers, cabbage, celery, kale, Brussels sprouts, mushrooms, zucchini, and fennel.

Fruits Low in Sugar

During an episode of sugar-craving, it's usually a good idea to pick low-sugar fruit items. Believe it or not, there are lots of those in the market! Just make sure to stock up on any of these: avocado, blackberries, raspberries, strawberries, blueberries, lime, lemon, and coconut. Also, note that tomatoes are fruits too, so feel free to make side dishes or dips with loads of tomatoes! Keep in mind that these fruits should be eaten fresh and not out of a can. If you do eat them fresh off the can, however, take a good look at the nutritional information at the back of the packaging. Avocadoes are particularly popular for those practicing the Ketogenic Diet because they contain LOTS of the good kind of fat.

Meat and Eggs

While some diets will tell you to skip the meat, the Ketogenic Diet encourages its consumption. Meat is packed with protein that will feed your muscles and give you a consistent energy source. It's a slow but sure burn when you eat protein as opposed to carbohydrates, which are burned faster and therefore stored faster if you don't use them immediately. But what kind of meat should you be eating? There's chicken, beef, pork, venison, turkey, and lamb. Keep in mind that quality plays a huge role here – you should be eating grass-fed organic beef or organic poultry if you want to make the most out of this food variety.

The organic option lets you limit the possibility of ingesting toxins in your body due to the production process of these products. Plus, the preservation process also means added salt or sugar in the meat, which can throw off the whole diet.

Nuts and Seeds

Nuts and seeds you should add in your cart include chia seeds, brazil nuts, macadamia nuts, flaxseed, walnuts, hemp seeds, pecans, sesame seeds, almonds, hazelnut, and pumpkin seeds. They also contain lots of protein and very little sugar, so they're great if you have the munchies. They're the ideal snack because they're quick, easy, and will keep you full. They're high in calories, though, which is why lots of people steer clear of them. As I mentioned earlier, the Ketogenic Diet has nothing to do with calories and everything to do with the nutrient you're eating. Don't pay too much attention to the calorie count, and just remember that they're a good source of fats and protein.

Dairy Products

Some people in their 50s already have a hard time processing dairy products, but for those who don't – you can happily add many of these to your diet. Make sure to consume sufficient amounts of cheese, plain Greek yogurt, cream butter, and cottage cheese. These dairy products are packed with calcium, protein, and a healthy kind of fat.

Oils

Nope, we're not talking about essentials oils but rather MCT oil, coconut oil, avocado oil, nut oils, and even extra-virgin olive oil. You can start using those for your frying needs to create healthier food options. The beauty of these oils is that they add flavor to the food, making sure you don't get bored quickly with the recipes. Try picking up different types of Keto-friendly oils to add some variety to your cooking.

Coffee and Tea

The good news is that you don't have to skip coffee if you're going on a Ketogenic Diet. The bad news is that you can't go to Starbucks anymore and order their blended coffee choices. Instead, beverages would be limited to unsweetened tea or unsweetened coffee to keep sugar consumption low. Opt for organic coffee and tea products to make the most out of these powerful antioxidants.

Dark Chocolate

Yes – chocolate is still on the menu, but it is limited to just dark chocolate. Technically, this means eating chocolate that is 70 percent cacao, which would make the taste a bit bitter.

Sugar Substitutes

Later in the recipes part of this book, you might be surprised at some of the ingredients required in the list. This is because while sweeteners are an important part of food preparation, you can't just use any kind of sugar in your recipe.

Remember: the typical sugar is pure carbohydrate. Even if you're not eating carbohydrates, if you're dumping lots of sugar in your food – you're not following the Ketogenic Diet principles.

So what do you do? You find sugar substitutes. The good news is that there are LOTS of those in the market. You can get rid of the old sugar and use any of these as a good substitute.

Stevia. This is perhaps the most familiar one in this list. It's a natural sweetener derived from plants and contains very few calories. Unlike your typical sugar, stevia may help lower the sugar levels instead of causing it to spike. Note, though, that it's sweeter than actual sugar, so when cooking with stevia, you'll need to lower the amount used. Typically, the ratio is 200 grams of sugar per 1 teaspoon of powdered stevia.

Sucralose. It contains zero calories and zero carbohydrates. It's an artificial sweetener and does not metabolize – hence the complete lack of carbohydrates. Splenda is a sweetener derived from sucralose. Note, though, that you don't want to use this as a baking substitute for sugar. Its best use is for coffee, yogurt, and oatmeal sweetening. Note that like stevia, it's also very sweet, it's 600 times sweeter than the typical sugar. Use sparingly.

Erythritol. It's a naturally occurring compound that interacts with the tongue's sweet taste receptors. Hence, it mimics the taste of sugar without actually being sugar. It does contain calories, but only about 5% of the calories you'll find in the typical sugar. Note, though, that it doesn't dissolve very well, so anything prepared with this sweetener will have a gritty feeling. This can be problematic if you're using the product for baking. As for sweetness, the typical ratio is 1 1/3 cup for 1 cup of sugar.

Xylitol. Like erythritol, xylitol is a type of sugar alcohol that's commonly used in sugar-free gum. While it still contains calories, the calories are just 3 per gram. It's a sweetener that's good for diabetic patients because it doesn't raise the body's sugar levels or insulin. The great thing about this is that you don't have to do any computations when using it for baking, cooking, or fixing a drink. The ratio of it with sugar is 1 to 1, so you can quickly make the substitution in the recipe.

What About Condiments?

Condiments are still on the table, but they won't be as tasty as you're used to. Your options include mustard, olive oil mayonnaise, oil-based salad dressings, and unsweetened ketchup. Of all these condiments, ketchup is the one with the most sugar, so make a point of looking for one with reduced sugar content. Or maybe avoid ketchup altogether and stick to mustard?

What About Snacks?

The good news is that there are packed snacks for those who don't have the time to make it themselves. Sugarless nut butters, dried seaweeds, nuts, and sugar-free jerky are all available in stores. The nuts and seeds discussed in a previous paragraph all make excellent snack options.

What About Labels?

Let's not fool ourselves into thinking that we can cook food every single day. The fact is that there will be days when there will be purchases for the sake of convenience. There are also instances when you'll have problems finding the right ingredients for a given recipe. Hence, you'll need to find substitutes for certain ingredients without losing the "Keto-friendly" vibe of the product.

So what should be done? Well, you need to learn how to read labels. Food doesn't have to be specially made to be keto-friendly. You just have to make sure that it doesn't contain any of the unfriendly nutrients or that the carbohydrate content is low enough.

Here's a step by step procedure on how to make a decision based on the labels:

1. First, take a good look at the ingredient list. You can usually find this at the bottom portion of the label and properly designated as "Ingredients."

2. The first step is to look at the sugar ingredient. If it's listed as one of the first five ingredients, that already means there's too much sugar in the product to be keto-friendly. Note, though, that sugar comes with many names. The words: glucose, fructose, maltose, lactose, dextrose, corn syrup, and more, are all indicative of sugar content. You'd want to make sure they're not listed within the first five ingredients of your buying food product. That's one of the best things about the food industry – they're required to list ingredients in the order of quantity so that the first ones listed have more volume in the product.

3. If the food passes the "sugar" test, you should next look at the carbohydrate content.

4. You'll notice that carbohydrates are often broken down into groups. Hence, labels may indicate that total carbohydrates are 5grams. Then right below that, you can see Dietary Fiber at 1gram and sugar at 1gram. The important thing to note here is that the dietary fiber and the sugar are part of the total carbohydrates.

5. Why is this important? Well, most people count the total carbohydrates when computing their carbohydrate consumption for the day. Hence, if your goal is to eat less than 50grams of carbohydrates during the day, then you'll be computing using the 5gram amount.

6. Some people, however, make use of the "net carbohydrates" when computing their consumption. Net carbohydrates are what you get when you subtract the other carbohydrate sources from the total carbohydrates. Hence, 5 grams less 1 gram for the fiber and another gram for sugar means that you'll have 3 grams of net carbohydrates.

7. Again – why is this important? The main distinction occurs for people who have diabetes. It's all about the insulin levels. However, it's all about the 50 grams of carbohydrates limitation in your diet. However, if you want to stay on the safe side, then counting the total carbohydrates is usually the best option.

CHAPTER 20:

Meal Plan

Days	Breakfast	Lunch/Dinner	Snacks
1	Almond, Coconut, Egg Wraps	Cauliflower Mac & Cheese	Chocolate Avocado Ice Cream
2	Bacon & Avocado Omelet	Mushroom & Cauliflower Risotto	Mocha Mousse
3	Bacon & Cheese Frittata	Pita Pizza	Strawberry Rhubarb Custard
4	Bacon& Egg, Breakfast Muffins	Skillet Tacos Cabbage	Creme Brulee
5	Bacon Hash	Taco Casserole	Chocolate Avocado Ice Cream
6	Bagels With Cheese	Creamy Salad Chicken	Mocha Mousse
7	Baked Apples	Spicy Keto Chicken Wings	Strawberry Rhubarb Custard
8	Baked EggsIn The Avocado	Cilantro and Lime Creamed Chicken	Creme Brulee
9	Banana Pancakes	Cheesy Quiche Ham	Pumpkin Pudding Pie
10	Breakfast Skillet	Loaded Cauliflower Rice	Vanilla Frozen Yogurt
11	Brunch BLT Wrap	Super Herbed Fish	Ice Cream
12	Cheesy Bacon & Egg Cups	Turkey Chili Avocado	Chocolate Avocado Ice Cream
13	Coconut Porridge Keto	Cheesy Shrimp, Tomato	Mocha Mousse

14	Cream Eggs Cheese	Cajun Chicken, Rosemary	Strawberry Rhubarb Custard
15	Creamy Basil, Baked Sausage	Sriracha Kabobs, Tuna	Creme Brulee
16	Almond, Coconut, Egg Wraps	Chicken Casserole Relleno	Pumpkin Pudding Pie
17	Bacon & Avocado Omelet	Steak Salad with Asian Spice	Chocolate Muffins
18	Bacon & Cheese Frittata	Chicken Chow Mein Stir Fry	Lemon Fat Bombs
19	Bacon & Egg Breakfast Muffins	Choy	Vanilla Frozen Yogurt
20	Bacon Hash	Buttery Garlic Steak	Mocha Mousse
21	Bagels With Cheese	Baked Lemon Salmon	Strawberry Rhubarb Custard
22	Baked Apples	One Sheet Fajitas	Creme Brulee
23	Baked Eggs In The Avocado	Balsamic Chicken	Pumpkin Pudding Pie
24	Banana Pancakes	CheesyKeto Meatballs	Chocolate Muffins
25	Breakfast Skillet	Beef Rib Steak with Parsley Lemon Butter	Lemon Fat Bombs
26	Brunch BLT Wrap	Marinated Flank Steak with Beef Gravy	Vanilla Frozen Yogurt
27	Cheesy Bacon & Egg Cups	Buttery Beef Loin and Cheese Sauce	Ice Cream
28	Coconut Keto Porridge	Chicken Wings Black Pepper with Sesame Seeds	Chocolate Avocado Ice Cream

Conclusion

Whether you have met your weight loss goals, your life changes, or you simply want to eat whatever you want again, here's the best way to come off the keto diet.

First, you need to prepare yourself mentally. You cannot just suddenly start consuming carbs again, for it will shock your system. Have an idea of what you want to allow back into your consumption slowly. Be familiar with portion sizes and stick to that amount of carbs for the first few times you eat post-keto. Start with non-processed carbs like whole grain, beans, and fruits. Start slow and see how your body responds before resolving to add carbs one meal at a time.

The things to watch out for when coming off keto are weight gain, bloating, more energy, and feeling hungry. The weight gain is nothing to freak out over, perhaps, you might not even gain any. It all depends on your diet, how your body processes carbs, and, of course, water weight. The length of your keto diet is a significant factor in how much weight you have lost, which is caused by the reduction of carbs. The bloating will occur because of the reintroduction of fibrous foods and your body getting used to digesting them again. The bloating van lasts for a few days to a few weeks. You will feel like you have more energy because carbs break down into glucose, which is the body's primary source of fuel. You may also notice better brain function and the ability to work out more.

www.ingramcontent.com/pod-product-compliance
Lightning Source LLC
Chambersburg PA
CBHW080622030426
42336CB00018B/3045